Current Topics in Microbiology and Immunology

149

Editors

Mechanisms in Myeloid Tumorigenesis 1988

Workshop
at the National Cancer Institute
National Institutes of Health
Bethesda, MD, USA, March 22, 1988

Organized and Edited by
G. L. C. Shen-Ong, M. Potter and
N. G. Copeland

With 42 Figures

Springer-Verlag
Berlin Heidelberg NewYork
London Paris Tokyo

Grace L. C. Shen-Ong, Ph. D.
Michael Potter, M. D.

Laboratory of Genetics
National Institutes of Health
National Cancer Institutes
Bethesda, MD 20892
USA

Neal G. Copeland, Ph. D.
Mammalia Genetics Laboratory
BRI - Basic Research Program
NCI - Frederick Cancer Research Facility
MD 21701
USA

ISBN-13: 978-3-642-74625-3 e-ISBN-13: 978-3-642-74623-9
DOI: 10.1007/978-3-642-74623-9

Library of Congress Catalog Card Number 15-12910

Softcover reprint of the hardcover 1st edition 1989

Printing: Color-Druck Dorfi GmbH, Berlin

2123/3020-543210

Preface

Through numerous discussions with colleagues it became apparent that the time was right to begin a series of workshop-like meetings on myeloid tumorigenesis. Myeloid tumors are the nonlymphocytic tumors of the hematopoietic system which include tumors of the neutrophilic, monocytic, erythrocytic, basophilic (mast cell) and megakaryocytic lineages.

Pioneering studies in myeloid tumorigenesis were initially made in chickens with the discovery of retroviruses that induce various kinds of myeloid tumors acutely (myelocytomatosis, myeloblastosis, and erythroblastosis). These avian retroviruses were subsequently shown to contain the oncogenes v-myb, v-ets, v-myc, v-erbA, or v-erbB.

There have been dramatic advances in studying the pathogenesis of hematopoietic tumors in genetically defined mammalian systems. Many of the well developed model systems in inbred mice, have focused on T- and B-lymphoma development. Although myeloid tumors have been found in mice, they have not been studied as intensively as lymphoid tumors. Possibly this is because myeloid tumors are less common than lymphoid tumors. Recently, there has been renewed interest in murine myeloid tumor systems. This focus has resulted from 1) the discovery of inbred strains of mice (e.g. BXH-2, AKXD-23, SJL/J) that are highly susceptible to spontaneous or induced myeloid tumorigenesis; 2) establishment of transplantable murine myeloid tumors (e.g. WEHI-3B, HAFTL-1, P388D1, ABML); 3) progress in culturing and propagating normal myeloid progenitor cells in vitro has been made possible by the use of purified growth factors or stromal cell feeder layers; and 4) the establishment of nontumorigenic factor-dependent cell lines (e.g. FDCP-1, 32D) for transformation studies. Several oncogenes that play a role in myeloid tumorigenesis in mice have been identified.

Concurrently, there have been exciting advances in finding a relatively high frequency of genetic lesions identified as nonrandom chromosomal rearrangements, deletions and amplifications in myeloid tumors in man [eg. $5q^-$, t(6;9), t(15;17), t(8;21), t(9;22)]. Emerging from these studies was the discovery of several oncogenes, most notably abl, that appear to play a role in myeloid tumor formation. Research in both the murine and human systems opens the possibilities for finding common underlying mechanisms in myeloid tumorigenesis in different species.

The common denominators in various forms of myeloid tumorigenesis may ultimately lie in the specific genes that are targets of mutagenesis. Consequently, we need to identify these common genes and determine how mutations in them influence the development of neoplasia. These and other questions form the basis for beginning this series of workshops. The first meeting was organized as a short, one day introduction (almost an impromtu meeting) that was held prior to the 6th Workshop on Mechanisms in B-cell Neoplasia in Bethesda, Maryland on March 22, 1988. We hope to continue the myeloid tumorigenesis meetings on a yearly basis.

The papers presented here, apologetically, do not encompass the entire field but do deal with many of the ongoing and leading problems in this area of research. The status of nonrandom chromosomal rearrangements in acute nonlymphocytic leukemia (ANLL) in man was discussed. Unlike the situation in man, there have been few reported examples of consistent cytogenetic changes in murine myeloid tumors. However, deletions in chromosome 2 have been observed in radiation-induced myeloid tumors of some inbred strains. A new protocol for inducing myeloid tumors in high frequency, which contain chromosome 2 deletions, is described here.

More progress has been made in identifying genes that are altered by retroviral integration in virally-induced myeloid tumors. In mice, a growing list of genes shown to be mutated by viral integration were described. These genes include the Myb, Fim-1, Fms (Fim-2), Evi-1 (Fim-3), and Evi-2 genes.

The in vitro culture of non-neoplastic myeloid precursor cells provides a valuable model system for studying myeloid tumorigenesis. It allows the induction of tumors and other abnormalities of growth in vitro. Much of this work has made use of transducing retroviruses, containing known oncogenes such as Myc and Raf. These viruses can transform myeloid progenitor cells in vitro.

We hope that the next workshop will focus in depth on genes that are involved in myeloid tumorigenesis and will begin, in a more mechanistic way, to explore the homologies and discordances that exist between human and mouse myeloid tumor systems. Only then will we be able to begin to formulate general mechanisms of myeloid tumorigenesis.

We are most grateful to the National Cancer Institute and NIH for sponsoring this meeting and for the organization assistance of CSR, Inc. We thank Ms. Victoria Rogers, LG, NCI, for assembling the manuscripts and preparing them for this publication.

Grace L.C. Shen-Ong, Ph.D.

and

Michael Potter, M.D.
National Cancer Institute
National Institutes of Health

and

Neal G. Copeland, Ph.D.
BRI - Basic Research Program
Frederick Cancer Research Facility

Table of Contents

List of Contributors

I. Classification of Myeloid Tumors

The Pathology of Murine Myelogenous Leukemias

Archibald S. Perkins

Department of Pathology, Brigham and Women's Hospital, 75 Francis Street, Boston, MA 02115

INTRODUCTION

Acute myelogenous leukemias (AML) can have a wide range of morphological variation, both in humans and in mice. Human AMLs have been divided into seven subtypes based on morphology of the leukemic cells and certain cytochemical reactions, which depend on the type of cellular differentiation and the degree of maturation (Bennett *et al.*, 1976, 1985). Correlation of these morphological subtypes with cytogenetic abnormalities has proved useful and interesting (Yunis *et al.*, 1984; Fourth International Workshop, 1984), while correlation with prognosis and response to treatment is less significant (Mertelsmann *et al.*, 1980). The finding of distinctive translocations in different subtypes argues that a) the subtypes are biologically distinct albeit related diseases with different antecedent leukemogenic events and b) mutation/alteration of gene(s) located at or near the translocation point is involved in the genesis of phenotype of the particular subtype to which the translocation is associated. The identification and characterization of genes significantly altered by the subtype-specific translocation should yield insight into both leukemogenesis and the control of normal differentiation. Indeed, identification of genes located at translocation breakpoints in human B and T cell neoplasms has yielded considerable insight into the transformation events leading to these tumors (Erikson and Croce, 1986; Tsujimoto and Croce, 1986).

Although radiation-induced murine myelogenous leukemias have a characteristic partial deletion of chromosome 2 (Resnitzky *et al.*, 1985; Hayata *et al.*, 1979), other common non-random chromosomal abnormalities have not been described in myelogenous leukemias of mice. Recently, however, the isolation of genes at common retroviral integration sites in virally-induced myelogenous leukemias has provided an important step towards a molecular understanding of myeloid differentiation and leukemogenesis (Buchberg *et al.*, 1988; Mucenski *et al.*, 1988; Sola *et al.*, 1986; Weinstein *et al.*; 1986; Gisselbrecht *et al.*, 1987; Bordereaux *et al.* 1987; Silver and Kozak, 1986). By analogy to the human myeloid tumors, one might expect a correlation to emerge between the genes altered by radiation damage or retrovirus insertion and the phenotype of the resultant myelogenous leukemia. For this reason, then, it is necessary to not only accurately establish the pathologic diagnosis of malignancy in experimental systems, but also to subclassify it, if possible, according to an accepted classification system, preferably one which is comparable to the accepted classification of human leukemias. Towards this end, I present a review of published cases of murine AML and attempt to categorize them on the basis of available information.

DIAGNOSIS OF MYELOGENOUS LEUKEMIA

In the human, the diagnosis of leukemia is based primarily on the findings from examination of peripheral blood smear, and bone marrow biopsy and aspirate. The criteria for the distinction between

Current Topics in Microbiology and Immunology, Vol. 149

Table 1. Features of human myelogenous leukemias

FAB	Type	Cytogenetics	Cytochemistry*	Morphology
M1	Myeloblastic without maturation	Variable	MP <3% CAE - NSE - LYSO -	Nongranular blasts, 1-3 nucleoli, few Auer rods
M2	Myeloblastic with maturation	t(8;21)	MP +/+++ CAE ++ NSE - LYSO +	Mix of myeloblasts and promyelocytes with azurophilic granules, bilobed or reniform nuclei and nucleoli
M3	Promyelocytic	t(15;17)	MP +++ CAE +++ NSE - LYSO +	Oval to reniform nuclei, abundant granular cytoplasm with clusters of Auer rods
M4	Myelomonocytic	inv (16) del (16)	MP +++ CAE + NSE + LYSO ++	Similar to M2 except promonocytes and monocytes exceed 20% in bone marrow
M5	Monocytic	t(9;11)	MP + NSE +++ LYSO +++	Can be poorly diff.(5A) with large blasts having lacy chromatin, nucleoli, abundant basophilie cytoplasm; can be differentiated (5B) with reniform or lobed nuclei

*Abbreviations: MP, myeloperoxidase; CAE chloracetate esterase; NSE, non-specific esterase; LYSO, lysozyme.

myelogenous and lymphoblastic leukemia, and the characteristics of the different subtypes are well described (Bennett *et al.*, 1976, 1985) (see Table 1). Usually, distinctive morphologic features of myeloid cells are seen on Wright-Giemsa or Romanowsky stained smears of peripheral blood or bone marrow blasts (e.g., the presence of granules or Auer rods in a moderately abundant cytoplasm, oval to reniform nuclei with finely granular chromatin and multiple nucleoli) (Kapff and Jandl, 1987). Cytochemical stains for myeloperoxidase and chloroacetate esterase can help identify granulocytic differentiation (Yam *et al.*, 1981), whereas monocytic differentiation is revealed by fluoride-inhibitable nonspecific esterase activity, best displayed using naphthyl butyrate as a substrate (Li, 1981).

Numerous monoclonal antibodies directed against human granulocytic and monocytic cell surface antigens have been developed (reviewed by Foon and Todd, 1986). These reagents are particularly useful for distinguishing myeloblasts from lymphoblasts (Griffin *et al.*, 1984; Herrmann *et al.*, 1983) and for identifying monocytic differentiation in myelomonocytic or monocytic leukemias (Ball *et al.*, 1983; Majdic *et al.*, 1981; Todd *et al.*, 1981). In general, studies of leukemic cells performed with monoclonal antibodies reveal considerable heterogeneity in the surface antigen expression of the leukemic cells from a given patient, and limited correlation between the morphologic subtype and the surface marker expression (Foon and Todd, 1986). Several genes encoding cell surface markers present on myeloid cells have been cloned, including CD 14 (Mo2, MY4) (Goyert et al., 1988), CD 33 (MY9) and CD 34 (MY10) (Simmonds and Seed, in press). These probes, or their murine counterparts, may prove helpful in analyzing murine myeloid tumors.

MURINE MYELOGENOUS LEUKEMIA

Diagnosis of myelogenous leukemia in the mouse rests primarily on autopsy findings. Premortem, the finding of myeloid blasts in the peripheral smear can be helpful (Dunn *et al.*, 1954), but bone marrow samples are difficult to obtain. Splenic enlargement, ruffling of the fur, pallor, and generalized weakness often are noted in the later stages of disease (Parsons *et al.*, 1962).

The spleen is invariably involved, weighing 3-15 times normal, and microscopically there is expansion of the red pulp and compression of the periarteriolar lymphoid tissue. Bone marrow involvement is variable and may depend on the stage of disease at autopsy. Findings in other organs are variable, as will be discussed below.

A variety of histopathologic types of myelogenous leukemias have been described in the mouse, induced by a number of agents including viruses, radiation, hormones, and carcinogens; also described are spontaneous myelogenous leukemias. Correlation to the human French-American-British (FAB) classification system (Bennett *et al.*, 1976) is usually possible on the basis of morphology, cytochemical reactions, and antibody staining of the leukemic cells. Cases of murine myelogenous leukemia described in the literature or reviewed by the author are described here and classified according to available information.

Table 2. Myelogenous leukemias in the mouse

Mouse Strain or Cell Line	Agent	Tumor Type	Reference and Incidence
LC wild mice, NIH Swiss	LC-MuLV	30% stem cell	Bryant *et al.*, 1981
C57BL/6	R-MuLV	Granulocytic leukemia	Boiron *et al.*, 1965
SJL/J	Radiation+ cortico-steroids	50-70% granulocytic leukemia	Resnitzky *et al.*, 1985
RFM C3H/He	Radiation	20-30% granulocytic leukemia	Hayata *et al.*, 1979
ICR/Ha	Thymectomy Rich MuLV	12% granulocytic leukemia	Siegler & Rich, 1967
C3H	Thymectomy Gross MuLV, passage A	13-20% granulocytic leukemia	Gross, 1960
NFS	Cas-Br-M MuLV	20-30% granulocytic leukemia 70-80% other	Frederickson, 1984
AKXD-23	Endogenous ecotropic MuLv	70% granulocytic leukemia	Mucenski *et al.*, 1986
DBA/2	F-MuLV	66% myeloblastic leukemia	Wendling *et al.*, 1983
C57BL/6	F-MuLV	52% nonthymic lymphomas, 20% granulocytic leukemias	Silver & Fredrickson, 1983

Table 2. Myelogenous leukemias in the mouse

Mouse Strain or Cell Line	Agent	Tumor Type	Reference
BXH-2	Ecotropic MuLV	100% myelomonocytic leukemia 100% of mice)	Bedigian *et al.*, 1984, Buchberg *et al.* (manuscript in preparation)
NIH Swiss mice	PyF101-Mo MuLV	45% lymphoblastic lymphoma, 54% myelomonocytic leukemia	Fan *et al.*, 1986
Bone marrow cells from C57BL/6-*bg/bg*	Cocultivation	Myelomonocytic leukemia	Naparstek, 1986
DBA/2	F-MuLV	87% Myelomonocytic leukemia	Shibaya and Mak, 1982
BALB/c	Pristane and *c-myc*	Monocyte/macrophage tumors	Baumbach, et al. 1987
BALB/c	Pristane & M-MuLV	Monocyte/macrophage tumors	Shen-Ong and Wolff, 1987

Stem Cell Leukemias

Dunn (1954) reviewed descriptions of stem cell leukemias by Engelbreth-Holm (1942), and Rask-Nielsen and Gormsen (1951). The leukemic cells were described as having morphologic features of both lymphoblasts and myeloblasts. More recent studies (Bryant *et al.*, 1981) have documented the occurrence of leukemias apparently arising in the spleens of Lake Casitas (LC)-MuLV-infected NIH Swiss mice or wild LC mice. They describe the leukemic cells as having large round vesicular nuclei, high nuclear to cytoplasmic ratio, diffuse heterochromatin, and prominent nucleoli. The cytoplasm, by light microscopy and electron microscopy was devoid of diagnostic myeloid or lymphoid features and routine cytochemistries were negative. In addition, immunofluorescence and immunoperoxidase studies with specific monoclonal antibodies failed to reveal B or T cell features (e.g., surface or cytoplasmic Ig, Thy 1). The early involvement of the splenic red pulp suggests this may be an early myelogenous leukemia (Fredrickson *et al.*, 1984). Similar tumors have been observed in mice inoculated with recombinant derivatives of Moloney-MuLV (Mo-MuLV) bearing alterations in the LTR (Pattengale, personal communication).

Myeloblastic Leukemia

In humans, the diagnosis of myeloblastic leukemia rests on finding a leukemic infiltrate of myeloid cells in the bone marrow which shows evidence of granulocytic differentiation. In the M1 subtype (acute myeloblastic leukemia without maturation), greater than 90% of the nonerythroid cells in the marrow are blasts which show one or more nucleoli, finely clumped chromatin, and either nongranular cytoplasm or a cytoplasm containing a few azurophilic granules or Auer rods. Greater than 3% of the blasts should be myeloperoxidase positive. Stains for nonspecific esterase may be positive, but are not inhibited by fluoride. In the M2 subtype, acute myeloblastic leukemia with maturation, or granulocytic leukemia, one finds significant maturation of the leukemic cells to or beyond the promyelocyte stage. The nuclei may be bilobed or reniform and typically contain nucleoli; cytoplasmic granules and Auer rods are frequent. In both these subtypes, monocytes account for less than 20% of the nonerythroid cells in the marrow.

In the mouse, both subtypes have been described, but a clear distinction between the two subtypes is not often made. These types have been found to occur in a number of mouse strains in response to a variety of agents, including: Inoculation of C57BL/6 or BALB/c mice with Rauscher (R-MuLV) virus (Boiron ***et al.***, 1965); irradiation of SJL/J (Fig. 1A and 1B), C3H/He or RFM (Fig. 1C) mice (Trakhtenbrot ***et al.***, in press; Resnitzky ***et al.***, 1985; Hayata ***et al.***, 1983; Upton ***et al.***, 1958); inoculation of MuLV into thymectomized mice (Siegler and Rich, 1967; Yokuro ***et al.***, 1964; Gross, 1960); inoculation of NFS mice with ecotropic MuLVs derived from Lake Casitas mice (Cas-Br-M and Cas2 Spl-MuLVs) (Fig. 1D) (Fredrickson ***et al.***, 1984; Holmes ***et al.***, 1986); inoculation of NIH Swiss mice with SRS-MuLV (Fig. 2A) (Fan ***et al.***, unpublished) and spontaneously in a proportion of AKXD-23 recombinant inbred mice (Fig. 2B) (Mucenski ***et al.***, 1986). The helper-independent component of the Friend virus complex has been reported to induce myeloblastic leukemias in DBA/2, C57BL/6, and [B6xC]F_1 strains, which are resistant to early erythroblastic disease (Wendling ***et al.***, 1983; Silver and Fredrickson, 1983; Chesebro ***et al.***, 1983). However, myelomonocytic leukemias arising in mice inoculated with cloned F-MuLV have also been reported (Shibuya and Mak, 1982; McGarry ***et al.***, 1974).

The presence of a leukemia is suggested by finding involvement of the splenic red pulp with compression or obliteration of the periarteriolar lymphoid zones in the spleen. The myelogenous nature of the infiltrate is indicated by cytologic features which include, reniform and ring-shaped nuclei, and scant to moderate eosinophilic cytoplasm suggesting granulocytic differentiation. The blasts, which often dominate the picture, show a high nuclear-to-cytoplasmic ratio, immature chromatin, and one to three nucleoli. The cytoplasm of the leukemic cells may be scant or difficult to visualize in the tissue infiltrates; touch preps and peripheral blood smears are helpful in allowing one to see a scant to moderate amount of eosinophilic, sometimes granular cytoplasm. Myeloperoxidase and chloroacetate esterase are positive in the leukemic cells. In addition, the tumors usually have germline configuration of immunoglobulin and T cell receptor genes (Mucenski ***et al.***, 1986), lack of phenotypic markers for T and B cells, and, in some series, the majority show immunoreactivity with the monoclonal antibody Mac-1 which stains the C3bi receptor (Holmes ***et al.***, 1985). Electron microscopic studies reveal features of early myeloid forms: nuclear euchromatin and one or more nucleoli, cytoplasmic polyribosomes and numerous mitochondria. Cytoplasmic granules are also present, more prominent in the more mature cells (Resnitzky ***et al.***, 1985).

The extent of leukemic infiltration into organs other than the spleen is variable. The radiation-induced myeloblastic leukemias in

SJL/J (Fig. 1A and 1B) and RFM (Fig. 1C) mice show a high mitotic rate with involvement of the lymph nodes, bone marrow, liver, and kidney (Fig. 2) as well as the spleen. In AKXD-23 mice (Fig. 2B) and in NFS mice inoculated with Cas2-Spl-M virus (Fig. 1D), tumor growth is limited to the red pulp of the spleen, the portal tracts of the liver, and, occasionally, the lymph nodes. Bone marrow involvement is less common (Fredrickson, personal communication). The degree of maturation of the leukemic cells may vary from one animal to another (within the same inbred strain) receiving the same agent, or within tissues of the same animal.

Two groups of tumors that fall into this morphologic category, the AKXD-23 myelogenous leukemias and the CasBrM-induced myelogenous leukemias in NFS mice, have been found to have retroviral integrations at the ***Evi-1*** locus (Mucenski ***et al.***, 1988). This locus, located on mouse chromosome 3, has recently been found to have sequence homology to a number of developmentally important genes that are DNA-binding proteins (Morishita ***et al.*** manuscript submitted). As of yet, there is no evidence that this gene is altered in the radiation-induced tumors. These latter tumors appear to have deletions of chromosome 2, involving region D through G (Resnitzky ***et al.***, 1985; Hayata ***et al.***, 1982). This appears to be a required yet not sufficient leukemogenic event, since 80% of irradiated SJL/J mice have chromosome 2 deletion at four months (Trakhtenbrot ***et al.***, in press), yet 50-70% of all irradiated mice develop AML with a mean latency of 300 days (Resnitzky ***et al.***, 1985).

<u>Acute Promyelocytic Leukemia</u>

This subtype (M3) accounts for 8% of human AML, and has distinctive features. Morphologically, >30% of the leukemic cells are promyelocytes. The cells have more abundant cytoplasm than M1 or M2 and have dense collections of azurophilic granules and bundles of Auer rods, which are strongly myeloperoxidase positive. This subtype has a characteristic translocation (t(15;17)) (Larson ***et al.***, 1984) which may involve the myeloperoxidase gene at the breakpoint (Weil ***et al.***, 1988). Clinical features include disseminated intravascular coagulation and a rapidly fatal outcome (Kantarjian ***et al.***, 1986).

A comparable disease in the mouse has not been well described. This may be due to the smaller size and fewer number of the primary azurophilic granules in murine granulocyte (Ogawa ***et al.***, 1983), features which make the murine promyelocyte stage less morphologically distinctive (Dunn, 1954). However, promyelocytic cell lines have been obtained from virally-induced murine leukemias (Ichikawa ***et al.***, 1976). Interestingly, some virally-induced leukemias in the BXH-2 mouse have retroviral insertions into the ***Evi-2*** locus (Buchberg ***et al.*** 1988b), which localizes to human chromosome 17 near the t(15;17) breakpoint seen in acute promyelocytic leukemia (M. LeBeau, personal communication). However, these tumors are typically myelomonocytic.

<u>Myelomonocytic Leukemia</u>

The leukemic cells of this subtype (M4) are morphologically heterogenous, and include blast forms (>30% of nonerythroid cells in the marrow), promonocytes, monocytes, as well as promyelocytes (Bennett ***et al.***, 1976). Monocytes typically exceed 20% of the nonerythroid cells in the bone marrow or peripheral blood. Morphologically, this subtype can be difficult to distinguish from the M2 subtype; the presence of monocytic cells must be confirmed by fluoride-inhibitable nonspecific esterase reaction (e.g., alpha-naphthyl butyrate esterase) (Bennett, ***et al.*** 1976, 1985). Monoclonal antibodies directed against monocyte-specific cell surface markers are particularly helpful in identifying AML subsets with monocytic differentiation (Foon and Todd, 1986). The myelomonocytic subtype accounts for 30% of human AML, and 25% of cases have an alteration of chromosome 16, either inversion or deletion (Yunis ***et al.***, 1984). Myelomonocytic leukemia (AMMoL) are well represented among murine AMLs. As with human cases, morphological identification of the monocytic components can be difficult and rests on cytochemical and immunoperoxidase studies.

Murine examples of AMMoL have been described by a number of investigators. A recombinant inbred mouse strain, BXH-2, has a 100% incidence of myeloid leukemia with an onset between 5-8 months (Bedigian ***et al.***, 1984). The tumors of this mouse (Fig. 2C and 2D) are aggressive, infiltrative myelomonocytic leukemias that involve multiple organs including bone marrow, peripheral blood, spleen, liver, lung, heart, muscle, kidney, and gastrointestinal tract. Cytology of the cells is best examined in the peripheral blood, where unclassifiable blast forms, early dysplastic monocytoid forms, and myeloid forms can be seen (Fig. 2D). The infiltrate in tissues is comprised of sheets of malignant cells with ovoid to reniform immature vesicular nuclei having characteristically clumped heterochromatin and one to three prominent nucleoli, and a scant amount of cytoplasm which is occasionally granular and eosinophilic (Fig. 2C). The cells stain for both nonspecific esterase and chloroacetate esterase, indicating both monocytoid and myeloid differentiation. The induction of the neoplasm appears to involve a horizontally-acquired ecotropic retrovirus. One common proviral integration site, present in 11% of mice with this tumor, has been identified, and host sequences from this locus have been cloned and localized to mouse chromosome 11 in a region with extensive homology to human chromosome 17 q12-21 (Buchberg ***et al.*** 1988a; M. LeBeau, personal communication). This is the region involved in t(15;17) observed in APML.

Fan ***et al.*** (1986) have described a myelomonocytic leukemia arising in NIH Swiss mice inoculated neonatally with a recombinant Mo-MuLV which contains a mutant polyoma enhancer inserted 5′ to the 75 bp repeats in the U3 region of the viral LTR (PyF101+Mo M-MuLV). The tumors arose in 5 of 11 animals, who died 14 weeks following inoculation. Six of 11 had lymphoblastic lymphoma, two of these concurrently with myelogenous leukemia. The myelomonocytic leukemic infiltrates were composed of "nonuniform pleomorphic populations of primitive cells with moderate amounts of cytoplasm and irregularly shaped nuclei...occasionally myelocytes and metamyelocytes were observed". The tumors involved the red pulp of the spleen and the paracortical regions of lymph nodes. A monocytic component to the leukemia was identified by positive immunoperoxidase studies with anti-Mac-2 antibody (See Table 3). This antibody, which can be used in paraffin-embedded tissues, reacts with a 32,000 mw cell-surface marker found on tissue-based macrophages, induced peritoneal macrophages, and Langerhas cells; granulocytes are reportedly negative (Flotte ***et al.***, 1983; Springer and Unkeless, 1984).

Table 3. Murine myeloid and monocytoid antigens defined by monoclonal antibodies

Antigen	Antigen M. W.*	Cellular Distribution	Reference
Mac-1	70kD 170kD	Macrophages histiocytes granulocytes NK cells; C3bi receptor	Springer and Unkeless 1984
Mac-2	32kD	Activated macrophages bronchial epithelium, kidney tubules, keratinocytes, epondyma	Springer and Unkeless 1984
Mac-3	100 - 170kD	Macrophages, granulocytes epithelial cells (liver, intestine) endothelial cells	Springer and Unkeless 1984
Ia	34kD	All B, monocytes	Holmes *et al.* 1986
8C5	?	Mature monocytes and inmature granulocytes	
FcR	47 - 70kD	Macrophages, neutrophilis B cells, some T cells; receptor for 1gG	Unkeless (1979)
F4/80	150kD	Mature macrophages, peripheral blood monocytes	Austyn and Gordon (1981)
GM 1.2	?	Granulocytes, macrophages	Shen and Boyse (unpublished)
GM 2.2		Mature granulocytes	Hibbs *et al.* 1984

*Molecular weight in kilodaltons (kD)

Moloney murine leukemia virus (Mo-MuLV) rarely if ever induces myelogenous leukemias; reason for the altered disease specificity of the PyF101+Mo M-MuLV recombinant virus is not clear.

Another interesting model of leukemogenesis has been described by Greenberger and coworkers. They have cocultivated murine growth factor-dependent bone marrow cells from C57BL/6J-***bg/bg*** mice (which have distinctive granulocyte morphology due to the beige (***bg***) mutation) with irradiated stromal cell lines (D2XR11), and following a period of 4 to 10 weeks of cocultivation have obtained factor-independent clones that were tumorigenic when injected into histocompatible mice. The tumor is comprised of primitive cells which occasionally exhibit a scant to moderate amount of eosinophilic granular cytoplasm and ringed or reniform nuclei (Fig. 3A). Myeloperoxidase stains were weakly positive, while alpha-naphthol chloroacetate esterase and naphthyl acetate esterase were strongly positive, indicating a myelomonocytic leukemia. The tumor infiltrated the spleen, bone marrow, and lymph nodes (Naparstek *et al.*, 1986).

Shibuya and Mak (1982) and McGarry *et al.* (1974) both described myelomonocytic leukemias in a number of mouse strains including DBA/2 and C57BL/6, which were inoculated neonatally with helper-independent F-MuLV. In 70% of F-MuLV-inoculated DBA-2 mice, Shibuya and Mak (1982) found a leukemia composed of myeloblasts and promonocytes in the spleen and peripheral blood; the leukemic cells stained for both alpha-naphthyl acetate esterase and peroxidase, indicating a myelomonocytic leukemia.

Monocytic Leukemia

In humans, the M5 subtype, monocytic leukemia (AMoL), is a malignant proliferation of monoblasts and promonocytes with varying numbers of monocytes (Fig. 3B). The leukemic cells are typically nonspecific esterase positive, which is inhibitable by fluoride (Bennett *et al.*, 1976). This is best demonstrated using naphthyl butyrate as a substrate (Li, 1981). By electron microscopy, the leukemic monoblasts show nuclear irregularity, nuclear blebs, perinuclear microfibrils (Freeman and Journey, 1971) and small peripheral lysosomal granules (O'Brien *et al.*, 1980). In humans, malignant neoplasms of the monocyte/macrophage lineage also include several solid tumors thought to be derived from tissue-based macrophages (e.g. histiocytes, Langerhans cells of the skin, and dendritic cells of the lymph nodes. These tumors include true histiocytic lymphoma, (Fig. 3C) and malignant histiocytosis (Jaffe, 1985) and represent malignant proliferations of tissue-based histiocytes rather than bone marrow-derived monocytes. Neither of these neoplasms has a leukemic phase. Human true histiocytic lymphomas are rare tumors, representing less than 2% of non-Hodgkin's lymphomas. They are rapidly growing, and give rise to bulky tumors in nodes, bone, or skin (van der Valk *et al.*, 1981; Willemze *et al.*, 1982) (Fig. 3C). Examples of monocytic leukemia in mice have not been described. However, several groups have described ascitic tumors comprised of clonal proliferations of malignant monocytic cells arising in the abdomen of mice pretreated with pristane and then inoculated with either Moloney-MuLV (Shen-Ong and Wolff, 1987) or a c-myc retrovirus (Baumbach *et al.*, 1986). The tumor-derived cell lines exhibit Mac1 and Mac2 antigens, as well as the Fc receptor. They contain nonspecific esterase, lysozyme, but not myeloperoxidase, and they exhibit phagocytosis. Necropsy of the mice reveals that the tumors are confined to the peritoneal cavity, and do not involve the spleen, liver, or bone marrow. Tumorigenesis is thought to involve the formation of pristane-induced oil granulomata and intraperitoneal extramedullary hematopoiesis followed by clonal acquisition of growth factor independence, perhaps by retrovirus insertion-mediated mutation of cellular growth factor genes or proto-oncogenes.

Murine "histiocytic" or "monocytic" sarcomas have been described (Furth and Furth, 1938; Gorer, 1946). Microscopically, the tumors were composed of infiltrations with cells resembling monocytes, with nuclei often "greatly elongated and narrow, frequently lobed and convoluted, assuming bizarre forms not seen in either lymphoid or myeloid leukemia. The cytoplasm stained red with eosin, was abundant and free from granules" (Furth and Furth, 1938). Occasionally the tumor infiltrate contained giant cells and eosinophils, giving the appearance of Hodgkin's disease. Dunn (1954) categorized this tumor as a reticulum-cell neoplasm Type A (RCS-A), grouping it together with diverse neoplasms in mice described by a number of investigators, based on morphology of the tumor cells on hematoxylin and eosin stained sections, rather than the cell of origin. RCS-A is a heterogeneous groups of tumors, which probably contains tumors which would be classified today as true histiocytic lymphomas, immunoblastic sarcomas, follicular center cell lymphomas, large cell type, or leiomyosarcomas depending on their histogenesis as discerned by immunoperoxidase studies, cytochemistries, and electron microscopy.

An interesting tumor with a morphologic similarity to RCS-A was found by Harris ***et al.*** (1988) to arise in 75% of transgenic mice containing the ***Ras*** oncogene under transcriptional control of the E-mu enhancer from the immunoglobulin heavy chain coupled to the SV40 promoter. This tumor (Fig. 3D) contains clusters of histiocytoid cells with fairly regular nuclei having coarsely granular chromatin and inconspicuous nucleoli, reminiscent of lymphocytic tumors. The abundant cytoplasm is faintly eosinophilic and finely granular. The cells are arranged in an almost organoid arrangement, an impression given by the circumscribing bands of connective tissue surrounding groups of cells. Mitoses are fairly frequent, and no evident phagocytosis is present. Multinucleated giant cells are not seen. The cells stain with anti-Mac-1 antibody (Harris, personal communication), which recognizes the C3bi receptor, present on macrophages, and histiocytes, and not found on epithelial cells of the kidney, lung, or skin (Flotte ***et al.***, 1983). While bearing a distinct resemblance to human true histiocytic lymphoma (Fig. 3D), strongly diagnostic features of histiocytic differentiation (van der Valk ***et al.***, 1981; Willemze ***et al.***, 1982) have not yet been demonstrated.

SUMMARY

Murine myelogenous leukemias can be classified into several distinct subgroups based on morphology, cytochemical staining, and immunoreactivity. The leukemias invariably involve the spleen and the extent of infiltration into other tissues is variable. The myelogenous nature of the leukemia is readily apparent in well-differentiated leukemias on the basis of morphology; with poorly differentiated leukemias, positive staining with chloroacetate esterase, nonspecific esterase, and certain monoclonal antibodies such as Mac-1, is helpful to establish myelogenous differentiation. Subgrouping of myelogenous leukemias depends on the presence or absence of monocytic differentiation, as ascertained by staining with Mac-2, electron microscopy or phagocytosis. Leukemias showing no monocytic differentiation can be classified as myeloblastic, corresponding to the FAB M1 and M2 subtypes in humans. Leukemias exhibiting both monocytic and granulocytic features are myelomonocytic, corresponding to the FAB M4 subtype. Tumors with only monocyte differentiation arise primarily as solid tumors in mice, and a leukemic phase is variable.

ACKNOWLEDGEMENTS

I thank Alan W. Harris, Paul K. Pattengale, Nechama Haran-Ghera, Torgny N. Fredrickson, Bruce A. Woda, Hung Fan, and Bernard Sass for contributing cases of murine leukemias. I also thank Janina

Longtine, David S. Weinberg, Phyllis C. Huettner, Herbert C. Morse III, Kevin L. Holmes and Neal G. Copeland for their helpful suggestions and comments.

REFERENCES

Austyn JM, Gordon S (1981) F4/80, a monoclonal antibody directed specifically against the mouse macrophage. Eur J Immunol 11: 805-815

Ball ED, Fanger MW (1983) The expression of myeloid-specific antigens on myeloid leukemia cells: Correlations with leukemia subclasses and implications for normal myeloid differentiation. Blood 61: 456-463

Baumbach WR, Keath EJ, Cole MD (1986) A mouse *c-myc* retrovirus transforms established fibroblast lines *in vitro* and induces monocyte-macrophage tumors *in vivo*. J Vir 59: 276-283

Bedigian HG, Johnson DA, Jenkins NA, Copeland NG, Evans R (1984) Spontaneous and inbred leukemias of myeloid origin in recombinant inbred BXH mice. J Virol 51: 586-594

Bennett JM, Catovsky D, Daniel MT, Flandrin G, Galton DAG, Gralnick HR, Sultan C (1976) Proposals for the classification of acute leukemia. Br J Haematol 33: 451-458

Bennett JM, Catovsky D, Daniel MT, Flandrin G, Galton DAG, Gralnick HR, Sultan C (1985) Proposed revised criteria for the classification of acute myeloid leukemia. A report of the French-American-British Cooperative Group. Ann Intern Med 103: 460-462

Boiron M, Levy J-P, Lasernet J, Oppenheim S, Bernard J (1965) Pathogenesis of Rauscher leukemia. J Natl Cancer Inst 35: 865-884

Bryant ML, Scott JL, Pal BK, Estes JD, Gardner MB (1981) Immuno-pathology of natural and experimental lymphomas induced by wild mouse leukemia virus. Am J Path 104: 272-282

Buchberg AM, Bedigian NG, Taylor BA, Brownell E, Ihle JN, Nagata S, Jenkins NA, Copeland NG (1988a) Localization of *Evi-2* to chromosome 11: Linkage to other proto-oncogene and growth factor loci using interspecific backcross mice. Oncogene Res 2: 149-165

Buchberg AM, Bedigian HG, Mucenski MM, Copeland NG, Jenkins NA (1988b) BXH-2 mice: A model system for identifying a new family of cellular oncogenes involved in myeloid leukemogenesis. Manuscript in preparation

Chesebro B, Portis JL, Wehrly K, Nishio J (1983) Effect of murine host genotype on MCF virus expression, latency, and leukemia cell type of leukemias induced by Friend murine leukemia helper virus. Virol 128: 221-233

Dunn T (1954) Normal and pathologic anatomy of the reticular tissue in laboratory mice with a classification and discussion of neoplasms. J Natl. Cancer Inst 14: 1281-1433

Engelbreth-Holm J (1942) Spontaneous and experimental leukemia in animals. Oliver & Boyd, Edinburgh

Erikson J, Croce CM (1986) The molecular genetics of human T cell leukemias and lymphomas. Curr Topics Microbiol Immunol 132: 175-182

Fan H, Mittal S, Chute H, Chao E, Pattengale PK (1986) Rearrangements and insertions in the Moloney murine leukemia virus alter biological properties *in vivo* and *in vitro*. J Virol 60: 204-214

Flotte TJ, Springer TA, Thorbecke GJ (1983) Dendritic cells and macrophage staining by monoclonal antibodies in tissue sections and epidermal sheets. Am J Path 111: 112-124

Foon KA, Todd RF III (1986) Immunologic classification and lymphoma. Blood 68: 1-31.

Fourth International Workshop on Chromosomes in Leukemia 1982 (1984) A prospective study of acute non-lymphocytic leukemia correlation of morphology and karyotype. Cancer Genet Cytogenet 11: 246-360

Fredrickson TN, Langdon WY, Hoffman PM, Hartley JW, Morse HC III (1984) Histologic and cell-surface antigen studies of hematopoietic tumors induced by Cas-Br-M murine leukemia virus. J Natl Cancer Inst 72: 447-454

Freeman AL, Journey LJ (1971) Ultrastructural studies on monocytic leukaemia. Br J Haematol 20: 225

Furth J, Furth OB (1938) Monocytic leukemia and other neoplastic diseases occurring in mice following intrasplenic injection of 1:2-benzpyrene. Am J Cancer 34: 169-183

Gorer PA (1946) The pathology of malignant histiocytoma (reticuloendothelioma) of the liver in mice. Cancer Res 6: 470-482

Goyert SM, Ferrero E, Rettig WJ, Yenamndra AK, Obata F, LeBeau MM (1988) The CD14 monocyte differentiation antigen maps to a region encoding growth factors and receptors. Science 239: 497-500

Griffin JD, Schlossman SF (1984) Expression of myeloid differentiation antigens in acute myeloblastic leukemia. Bernard A, Baumsell L, Dausset J, Milstein C, Schlossman JF (eds); Leukocyte Typing. Springer Verlag, New York, p. 404

Gross L (1960) Development of myeloid (chloro-)leukemia in thymectomized C3H mice following inoculation of lymphatic leukemia virus. Proc Soc Exp Biol Med 103: 509-514

Harris AW, *et al*. (1988) Manuscript in preparation.

Hayata I, Ishihara T, Hirashima K, Sado T, Yamagiwa J (1979) Partial deletion of chromosome #2 in myelocytic leukemias of irradiated C3H/He and RFM mice. J Natl Cancer Inst 63: 843-848

Hayata I, Seki M, Yoshida K, Hirashima K, Sado T, Yamagiwa J, Ishihara T (1983) Chromosomal aberrations observed in 52 mouse myeloid leukemias. Cancer Res 43: 367-373

Herrmann F, Komischke B, Odenwald E, Ludwig WD (1983) Use of monoclonal antibodies as a diagnostic tool in human leukemia: I. Acute myeloid leukemia and acute phase of chronic myeloid leukemia. Blut 47: 157-163

Hibbs ML, Hogarth PM, Scott BM, Harris RA, McKenzie IFC (1984) Monoclonal antibody to murine neutrophils: identification of the Gm-2.2 specificity. Immunol 133: 2619-2623

Holmes KL, Palaszynski E, Fredrickson TN, Morse HC III, Ihle JN (1985) Correlation of cell-surface phenotype with the establishment of interleukin 3-dependent cell lines from wild-mouse murine leukemia virus-induced neoplasms. Proc Natl Acad Sci USA 86: 6687-6691

Holmes KL, Langdon WY, Fredrickson TN, Coffman RL, Hoffman PM, Hartley JW, Morse HC III (1986) Analysis of neoplasms induced by Cas-Br-M MuLV extracts. J Immunol 137: 679-688

Ichikawa Y, Maeda M, Horivchi M (1976) ***In vitro*** differentiation of Rauscher-virus-induced myeloid leukemia cells. Int J Cancer 17: 789-797

Jaffe ES (1985) Malignant histiocytosis and true histiocytic lymphomas. In Surgical pathology of lymphnodes and related organs. WB Saunders, Philadelphia, p. 381-411

Kantarjian HM, Keating MJ, Walters RS, Estey EH, McCredie KB, Smith TL, Dalton WT Jr, Cork A, Trujillo JM, Freiveich EJ (1986) Acute promyelocytic leukemia. MD Anderson hospital experience. Am J Med 80: 789-797

Kapff C, Jandl JH (1981) Blood: Atlas and sourcebook of hematology. Little Brown & Co., Boston, p. 92

Larson RA, Kondo K, Vardiman JW, Butler AE, Golomb HM, Rowley JD (1984) Evidence for a 15:17 translocation in every patient with acute promyelocytic leukemia. Am J Med 76: 827-841

Li CY (1981) Chapter 9 in Current Hematology, Vol. 1, Fairbanks VF (ed.) John Wiley & Sons, New York

Linch DC, Allen C, Beverley PCL, Bynoe AG, Scott CS, Hogg N (1984) Monoclonal antibodies differentiating between monocytic and non-monocytic variants of AML. Blood 63: 566-573

Majdic O, Bettelheim P, Stockinger H, Aberer W, Liszka K, Lutz D, Knapp W (1984) M2, a novel myelomonocytic cell surface antigen and its distribution on leukemic cells. Int J Cancer 33: 617-623

McGarry MP, Steeves RA, Eckner RJ, Mirand EA, Trudel PJ (1974) Isolation of a myelogenous leukemia inducing virus from mice infected with the Friend virus complex. Int J Cancer 13: 867-878

Morishita K, Parker DS, Mucenski ML, Jenkins NA, Copeland NG, Ihle JN (1988) Retroviral activation of a novel gene encoding a zinc finger protein in IL-3 dependent myeloid leukemia cell lines. Manuscript submitted.

Mertelsmann, R, Thaler HT, To L, Gee TS, McKenzie S, Schauer P, Friedman A, Arlin Z, Cirrincione C, Clarkson B (1981) Morphological classification, response to therapy, and survival in 263 adult patients with acute nonlymphoblastic leukemia. Blood 56: 773-781

Mucenski ML, Taylor BA, Jenkins NA, Copeland NG (1986) AKXD recombinant inbred strains: Models for studying the molecular genetic basis of murine lymphomas. Mol Cell Biol 6: 4236-4243

Mucenski ML, Taylor BA, Ihle JN, Hartley JW, Morse HC III, Jenkins NA, Copeland NG (1988) Identification of a common ecotropic viral integration site, *Evi-1*, in the DNA of AKXD murine myeloid tumors. Mol Cell Biol 8: 301-308

Naparstek E, FitzGerald TJ, Sakakeeny MA, Klassen V, Pierce JH, Woda BA, Flaco J, Fitzgerald S, Nizin P, Greenberger JS (1986) Induction of malignant transformation of cocultivated hematopoietic stem cells by x-irradiation of murine bone marrow stromal cells *in vitro*. Cancer Res 46: 4677-4684

O'Brien M, Catovsky D, Costello C (1980) Ultrastructural cytochemistry of leukemic cells: characterization of the early small granules of monoblasts. Br J Haematol 45: 201-208

Ogawa T, Koerten HK, Brederoo P, Daems WTH (1983) A comparative study of primary and secondary granules in monocytopoiesis and myelopoiesis of mouse bone marrow. Cell Tiss Res 228: 107-115

Parsons DF, Upton AC, Bender MA, Jenkins VK, Nelson ES, Johnson RR (1962) EM observations on primary serially passaged radiation-induced myeloid leukemias of the RF mouse. Cancer Res 22: 728-736

Rask-Nielsen R, Gormsen H (1951) Spontaneous and induced plasma-cell neoplasia in a strain of mice. Cancer 4: 387-397

Resnitzky P, Estroz Z, Haran-Ghera N (1985) High incidence of acute myeloid leukemia in SJL/J mice after x-irradiation and corticosteroids. Leuk Res 9: 1519-1528

Scheid MP, Triglia D (1979) Further description of the Ly-5 system. Immunogenetics 9: 423-433

Shen-Ong GLC, Wolff L (1987) Moloney murine leukemia virus-induced myeloid tumors in adult BALB/c mice: Requirement of *c-myb* activation but lack of *v-abl* involvement. J Virol 61: 3721-3725.

Shibuya T, Mak TW (1982) Host control of susceptibility to erythroleukemia and to the types of leukemia induced by the Friend MLV: Initial and late stages. Cell 31: 483-493

Siegler R, Rich MA (1967) Pathogenesis of virus-induced myeloid leukemia in mice. J Natl Cancer Inst 38: 31-50

Silver JE, Fredrickson TN (1983) Susceptibility to Friend helper virus leukemias in CXB recombinant inbred mice. J Exp Med 158: 1693-1702

Springer TA, Unkeless JC (1984) Analysis of macrophage differentiation and function with monoclonal antibodies. Contemp Topics Immunobiol 13: 1-31

Sola B, Fichelson S, Bordereaux D, Tambourin, Gisselbrecht S (1986) ***Fim-1*** and ***Fim-2***: Two new integration regions of Friend MuLV in myeloblastic leukemias. J Virol 60: 718-725

Trakhtenbrot L, Krauthgamer R, Resnitzky P, Haran-Ghera N (1988) Deletion of chromosome 2 is an early event in the development of radiation-induced myeloid leukemias in SJL/J mice. Leukemia In press

Tsujimoto Y, Croce CM (1986) Molecular genetics of human B-cell eonplasia. Curr Top Microbiol Immunol 132: 183-192

Unkeless J (1979) Characterization of a monoclonal antibody directed against mouse macrophage and lymphocyte Fc receptors. J Exp Med 150: 580-596

Upton AC, Wolff FF, Furth J, Kimball AW (1958) A comparison of the induction of myeloid and lymphoid leukemias in X-radiated RF mice. Cancer Res 18: 842-848

van der Valk P, te Velde J, Jansen J, Ruiter DJ, Spaander PJ, Cornelisse CJ, Meijer CJ (1981) Malignant lymphoma of true histiocytic origin: Histiocytic sarcoma. A morphological, ultrastructural, immunological, cytochemical and clinical study of 10 cases. Virch Arch A 391: 249-265

Weil SC, Rosner GL, Reid MS, Chishom RL, Lemons RS, Swanson MS, Carrino JJ, Diaz MO, LeBeau MM (1988) Translocation and rearrangement of myeloperoxidase gene in acute promyelocytic leukemia. Science 240: 790-792

Weinstein Y, Ihle JN, Lavu S, Reddy EP (1986) Truncation of the ***c-myb*** gene by a retroviral integration in an interleukin 3-dependent myeloid leukemia cell line. Proc Natl Acad Sci USA 83: 5010-5014

Wendling F, Fichelson S, Heard JM, Gisselbrecht S, Varet B, Tambourin P (1983) Induction of myeloid leukemias in mice by biologically cloned ecotropic F-MuLV. In Scolnick E, Levine E (eds) Tumor viruses and differentiation. Alan R. Liss, New York, p. 357-362

Willemze R, Ruiter DJ, van Vloten WA, Meijer CJLM (1982) Reticulum cell sarcoma (large cell lymphomas) presenting in the skin. High frequency of true histiocytic lymphoma. Cancer 50: 1367-1379

Yam LT, Li CY, Crosby WH (1971) Cytochemical identification of monocytes and granulocytes. Am J Clin Path 55: 283-290

Yokuro K, Takemoto H, Kunii A (1964) Role of mouse lymphoma virus in induction of myeloid leukemia by x-ray. Ann NY Acad Sci 114: 203-212

Yunis JJ (1984) High-resolution chromosomes as an independent prognostic indicator in adult acute nonlymphocytic leukemia. New Engl J Med 311: 812-818

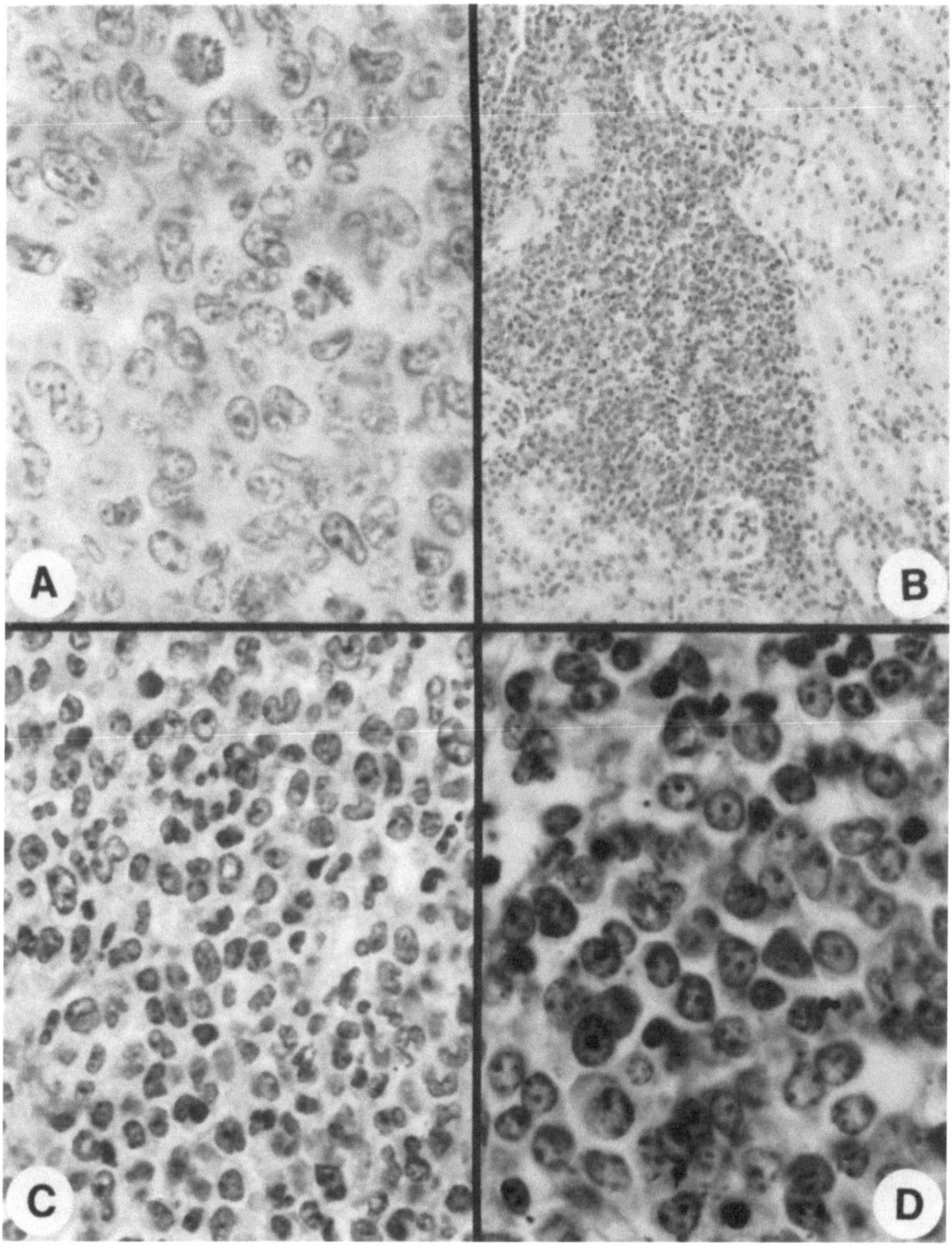

Figure 1: Irradiated SJL/J mouse, spleen (A) and kidney (B); irradiated RFM mouse, spleen (C); Cas 2 Spl MuLV-inoculated NFS mouse, spleen (D). A, C, D, original magnification 100x. B, original magnification, 10x.

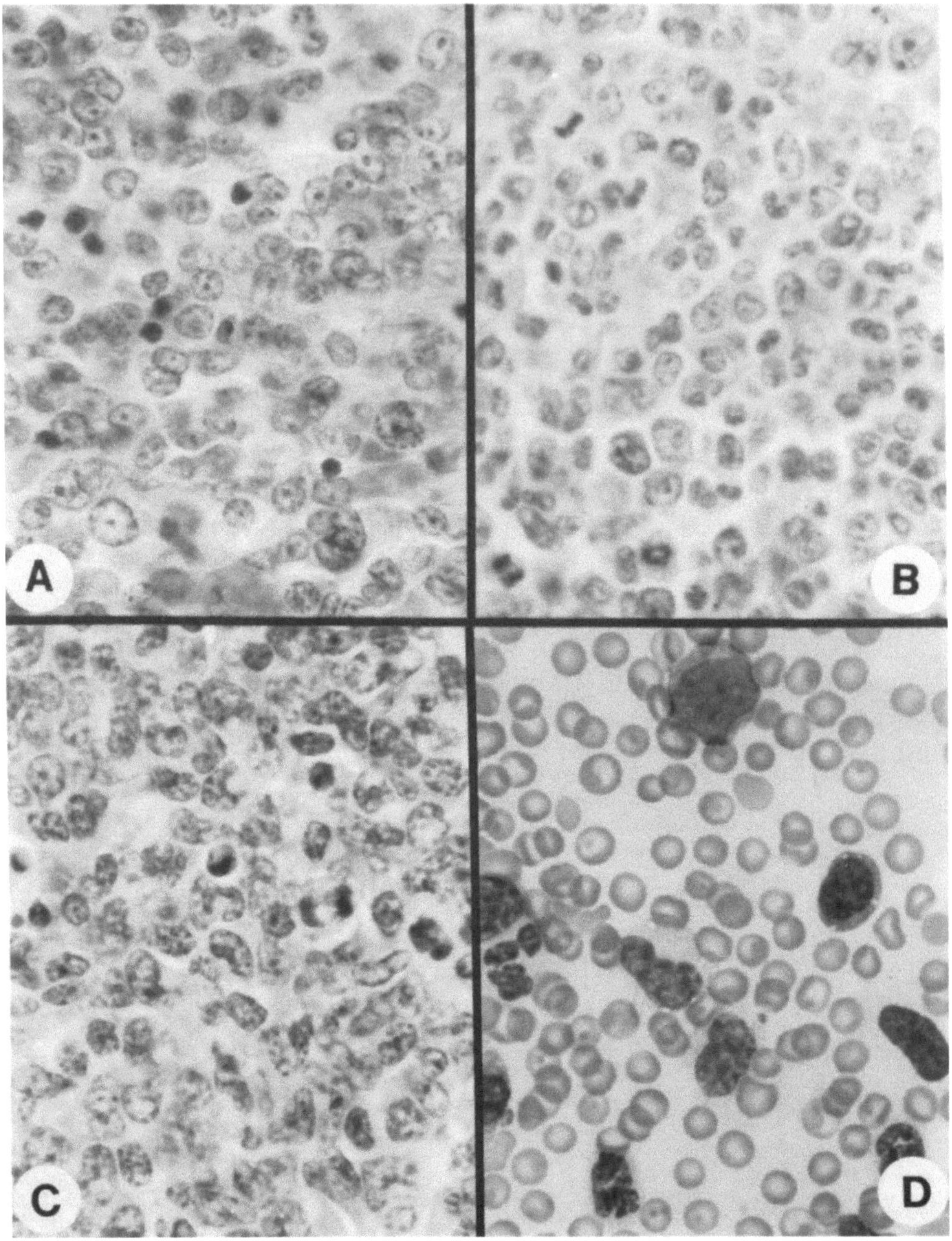

Figure 2: NIH Swiss mice inoculated with SRS-MuLV, spleen (A); AKXD-23 mouse, spleen (B); BXH-2 mouse, spleen (C) and peripheral blood (D). Original magnification, 100x.

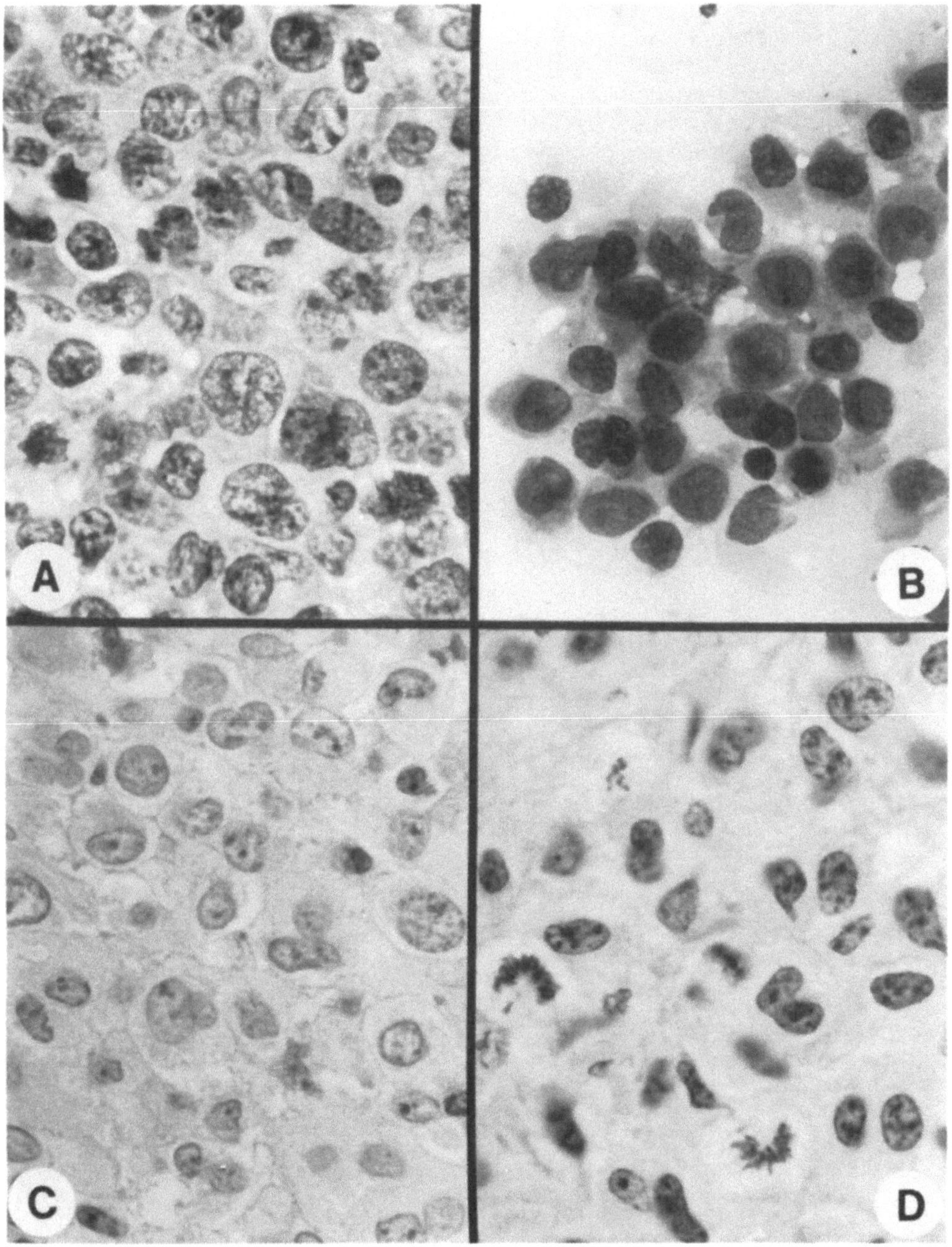

Figure 3: Tumor derived from C57BL/6-***bg/bg***, factor-independent bone marrow cells (A); human acute monocytic leukemia, touch prep of spleen (B); human true histiocytic lymphoma (C); Eμ-SV-ras-induced tumor (D). Original magnification, 100x.

II. Specific Chromosomal Abnormalities in Human and Murine Myeloid Hematologic Malignancies

Chromosomal Abnormalities in Myeloid Hematologic Malignancies

C.M. Rubin and M.M. Le Beau

Section of Pediatric Hematology/Oncology, Department of Pediatrics and Joint Section of Hematology/Oncology, Department of Medicine, The University of Chicago, 5841 S. Maryland Ave., Box 97, Chicago, IL 60637

INTRODUCTION

In the majority of patients with myeloid hematologic malignancies, the neoplastic cells have acquired clonal chromosomal abnormalities. A number of specific cytogenetic abnormalities have been recognized that are very closely, and often uniquely, associated with morphologically and clinically distinct subsets of these diseases. The detection of one of these recurring abnormalities can be quite helpful in establishing the correct diagnosis and can add information of prognostic importance. In addition, the appearance of new abnormalities in the karyotype of a patient under observation often signals a change in the pace of the disease, usually to a more aggressive disorder.

The precise role of chromosomal abnormalities in the pathogenesis or perpetuation of malignant clones is unknown. However, data obtained recently from the molecular analyses of the DNA sequences that are located at the sites of the breaks in recurring translocations, or within chromosomal segments that are deleted, suggests that these genes play an integral role in the process of malignant transformation. Whether the observed chromosome abnormality is the primary event in malignant transformation or a secondary manifestation of clonal expansion is not clear. It seems likely that genetic aberrations not detectable by cytogenetic techniques using light microscopy may be present in those patients whose malignant cells appear to have a normal karyotype. Thus, cytogenetic analysis can provide information of clinical importance as well as contribute to our understanding of the fundamental genetic changes in cells which give rise to these neoplasms.

We review the chromosomal abnormalities that are associated with the myeloid hematologic diseases, including the chronic myeloproliferative disorders (MPD), myelodysplastic syndromes (MDS), and acute nonlymphocytic leukemia (ANLL). MPD includes chronic myelogenous leukemia (CML), polycythemia vera (PV), essential thrombocythemia (ET) and myelofibrosis with myeloid metaplasia (MMM). Primary or de novo MDS and ANLL are considered according to the classification schemas devised by the French-American-British Cooperative Group (FAB). Secondary or therapy-related MDS and ANLL are discussed in a separate section. Complete references for the material presented here may be found in Le Beau and Larson (1988). Relevant additional reading is included in the reference section.

Current Topics in Microbiology and Immunology, Vol. 149

CHRONIC MYELOPROLIFERATIVE DISORDERS

Chronic Myelogenous Leukemia

Chronic phase: CML is a particularly important subtype of leukemia because it was in this disease that the first consistent chromosomal abnormality in a malignant disease was noted. This abnormality, the Philadelphia or Ph^1 chromosome, was first described in 1960 by Nowell and Hungerford as a deletion of part of the long arm of a G-group chromosome. The nature of the chromosomal aberration was clarified in 1973, when Rowley reported that the Ph^1 chromosome resulted from a reciprocal translocation involving chromosomes 9 (break at band q34) and 22 (break at band q11). Studies with chromosomal polymorphisms have shown that in a particular patient the same chromosome 9 (or 22) of each homologous pair is involved in the rearrangement in all of the malignant cells. These observations confirm earlier work based on enzyme markers, indicating that the CML cells originated from a single cell and were therefore clonal in origin.

Historically, about 85% of patients diagnosed as having CML were found to have the Ph^1 chromosome. Identification of patients as Ph^1-positive (Ph^1+) or Ph^1-negative (Ph^1-) was found to be clinically significant in that Ph^1+ patients had a better prognosis than did those patients with Ph^1- CML (42 vs. 15 months survival). Patients with a Ph^1 chromosome and additional chromosomal abnormalities (1-30% of patients examined at initial diagnosis during the chronic phase) have not had a substantially poorer survival rate in some series than those patients who have only a Ph^1 chromosome. A change in the karyotype, however, is considered to be a grave prognostic sign indicating progression to the acute blast phase; the usual duration of survival after such a change is 2-5 months.

Recently, evidence has accumulated which suggests that CML should be defined by the presence of the Ph^1 chromosome, and that patients without this abnormality should be considered to have a different disorder. Careful review of patients initially diagnosed as having CML but whose cells lack the Ph^1 chromosome shows that most of these patients have some type of myelodysplastic syndrome (MDS), most commonly chronic myelomonocytic leukemia or refractory anemia with excess blasts. The most common abnormality in these patients is trisomy 8. These observations suggest that, with very few exceptions, Ph^1- CML does not exist. The absence of the Ph^1 chromosome thus raises the suspicion that the patient actually has a myelodysplastic syndrome or a myeloproliferative disorder other than CML. It is notable, however, that the leukemia cells in rare individual cases which lack the Ph^1 chromosome appear to contain a DNA rearrangement, in which the molecular consequences are identical to that of the t(9;22) (described below).

The karyotypes of many Ph^1+ patients with CML have been examined with banding techniques by a number of investigators; the 9;22 translocation was identified in 92% of Ph^1+ patients. The remaining patients had variant translocations. Until very recently, these were thought to be of two kinds: one appeared to be a simple translocation involving chromosome 22 and a chromosome other than 9 and the other was a complex translocation involving three or more chromosomes, two of which were chromosomes 9 and 22. Recent data clearly demonstrate that chromosome 9 is affected in the simple as well as in the complex translocations, and that previously its involvement had been overlooked. Thus, all variant translocations in CML can be considered to be complex translocations.

Molecular analysis of the DNA sequences that are located at the chromosomal breakpoints of both the standard and variant translocations in CML has revealed that the proto-oncogene ABL is consistently translocated adjacent to a region of a gene (BCR) on chromosome 22, known as the breakpoint cluster region (bcr). This translocation results in the formation of a chimeric gene which contains protein coding sequences from both the ABL and BCR genes. The consequence of this translocation is the production of a larger fusion protein (210 kilodaltons) that has high tyrosine kinase activity. Several lines of evidence suggest that this BCR/ABL fusion protein plays a role in the transformation of myeloid cells. Recently, analysis of leukemia cells from rare patients with CML who lack the Ph^1 chromosome has revealed a rearrangement involving ABL and BCR that is detectable only at the molecular level. This provides further evidence that the t(9;22) and subsequent fusion of the ABL and BCR genes is characteristic of virtually all CML cases.

Acute phase: As they enter the terminal acute phase (blast crisis) of CML, most patients (80%) show karyotypic evolution with the appearance of new chromosomal abnormalities in very distinct patterns in addition to the Ph^1 chromosome. For this reason, cytogenetic studies may be useful in confirming the clinical impression of the accelerated or acute phase of the disease. A change in the karyotype is considered to be a grave prognostic sign. The available data suggest that with the exception of an isochromosome of the long arm of chromosome 17 [i(17q)], which is usually associated with a myeloid type of blast transformation, there is no association of a particular karyotype with the lymphoid or with the myeloid type of blast transformation, and that these additional abnormalities are not correlated with the response to therapy during the acute phase. The most common changes, a gain of chromosomes 8 or 19, or a second Ph^1, and an i(17q), frequently occur in combination to produce modal chromosome numbers of 47-50.

Polycythemia Vera

PV is the second most extensively studied MPD. Of untreated and treated PV patients (excluding patients analyzed only in the leukemic blast phase), one-fourth (23%) have chromosomally abnormal clones in their initial analysis. Abnormalities are less common in untreated patients than in those who have been treated with cytotoxic agents prior to their first cytogenetic examination (14% versus 39%, respectively). The incidence of abnormal clones is even higher (85%) in treated PV patients whose disease has transformed to a leukemic phase.

In PV, the presence of cytogenetic abnormalities at diagnosis does not necessarily predict a short survival or the development of leukemia. An evolutionary change in the karyotype during the disease course, however, may be an important sign of transformation to leukemia.

In the polycythemic phase of PV, the nonrandom distribution of chromosomal changes is particularly evident in the gain of chromosomes, which usually involves chromosomes 8 (15%) or 9 (20%). It is notable that a number of patients with PV show gains of both No. 8 and No. 9; clones containing both +8 and +9 are seldom observed in other hematologic diseases and, thus, may be unique to PV. With respect to structural rearrangements, chromosomes 20 (35%) and 1 (20%) are the most frequently rearranged chromosomes noted in PV. In particular, a deletion of the long arm of chromosome 20, most commonly del(20)(q11.2q13.3), is observed in approximately 30% of patients with PV. Although initially thought to be diagnostic of PV, a del(20q) has also been observed in ANLL, MDS, and other MPD. Most of the reported abnormalities of chromosome 1 in PV have consisted of trisomy of all or part (1q21-qter) of the long arm (15% of patients). As in the del(20q) abnormality, these rearrangements are not specific for PV. Trisomy of 1q, especially of bands 1q25-q32 and 1q23-q25, occur frequently both in hematologic diseases as well as in solid tumors.

The cytogenetic patterns of the malignant cells in PV patients who have developed ANLL show some similarities to those observed in the polycythemic phase, e.g., +8, +9, del(20q), but there are certain striking differences as well. For example, loss of number 7 is rarely observed in the polycythemic phase but is seen in 20% of patients in the leukemic phase. Rearrangements of chromosome 5, particularly a del(5q), are the most frequent changes noted in advanced disease (40% of patients). As described in a later section, abnormalities of chromosomes 5 and/or 7 are the most common abnormalities noted in therapy-related ANLL, suggesting that the leukemia in some patients with PV may have a similar etiology. It has been shown that the chronic use of oral alkylating agents such as chlorambucil or the use of P^{32} during the chronic phase of PV significantly increases the rate of transformation to leukemia.

Essential Thrombocythemia

Definite chromosomal abnormalities have been found in only 5% of patients. The data currently available do not reveal consistent karyotypic abnormalities in ET.

Myelofibrosis with Myeloid Metaplasia

Cytogenetic analysis of bone marrow cells of patients with MMM has revealed the presence of clonal abnormalities in 35% of patients. In general, these abnormalities are similar to those noted in other malignant myeloid disorders. The most common anomalies are trisomy 8, loss of chromosome 7 or a del(7q), and deletions of the long arms of chromosomes 11 and 20. More recently, a recurring deletion of the long arm of chromosome 13 has been reported in patients with MMM as well as with other malignant myeloid disorders. In these rearrangements, the consistently deleted band is 13q14. Similar to CML and PV, a change in the karyotype in MMM may signal evolution to acute leukemia.

PRIMARY MYELODYSPLASTIC SYNDROMES

Several laboratories have reported that clonal chromosomal abnormalities can be detected in bone marrow cells in 40-70% of patients with primary MDS at the time of diagnosis. This contrasts with the 70-95% incidence of cytogenetic abnormalities detected in patients with ANLL de novo. Although trisomy 8 and loss of all or part of the long arm (q arm) of chromosomes 5 or 7 are common in both disorders, the specific structural rearrangements that are closely associated with distinct morphologic subsets of ANLL de novo described below are almost never seen in MDS. With several exceptions (such as the 5q- syndrome), chromosomal abnormalities in MDS have not correlated with specific clinical or morphological subsets using the criteria of the French-American-British (FAB) group.

Patients with MDS may have single or multiple chromosome changes. A single chromosome change involves a single numerical change or a structural abnormality involving only one chromosome or a balanced translocation involving only two chromosomes. Occasionally, several unrelated abnormal clones may be detected; the frequency of such unrelated clones may be higher than that observed in ANLL de novo. Additional chromosomal aberrations may evolve during the course of MDS or an abnormal clone may emerge in a patient with a previously normal karyotype; these changes appear to portend transformation to leukemia.

The ability of cytogenetic analysis to predict the outcome for any individual patient with MDS is made more difficult because MDS is a life-threatening disorder due to persistent and profound pancytopenia (marrow failure), regardless of whether transformation to acute leukemia occurs. Thus, the presence of chromosomal abnormalities has not correlated with survival in several large series. However, the presence of an abnormal clone at diagnosis has correlated with the evolution of leukemia.

The 5q- syndrome is a distinctive hematological disorder which occurs primarily in older women. In contrast to other MDS where males predominate, the male:female ratio here is 0.5. Eighty percent of patients with the primary 5q- syndrome are older than 50 years. Patients present with a refractory macrocytic anemia and normal or elevated platelet counts. The marrow is characterized by the presence of monolobulated and bilobulated micromegakaryocytes. Approximately two-thirds of patients have less than 5% blasts in the marrow (RA or refractory anemia with ringed sideroblasts, RARS) and the remainder have RAEB. Although 75% of cases have a del(5)(q13q33), other interstitial deletions [del(5)(q15q33) or del(5)(q22q33)] may be present. These patients can have a relatively benign course which extends over several years.

ACUTE NONLYMPHOCYTIC LEUKEMIA DE NOVO

There have now been numerous reports describing cytogenetic analyses of relatively large series of unselected patients with ANLL as well as of single cases of selected patients. In earlier series, abnormal karyotypes were reported in approximately 50% of all patients with ANLL de novo whose bone marrow cells were examined with banding techniques. The detection of cytogenetic abnormalities increases markedly when techniques for culturing leukemia cells and for obtaining prophase and prometaphase chromosomes are used. Currently, we are detecting an abnormal clone in 85% of ANLL patients. The most frequent abnormalities are a gain of chromosome 8 and a loss of chromosome 7; these are seen in most subtypes of ANLL, although there are some interesting differences in frequency. Initially, it appeared that ANLL patients with a normal karyotype had a significantly longer survival than those with any detectable chromosomal abnormality. More recently, it has become clear that the prognostic importance resides within specific chromosome changes, several of which are associated with higher response rates and longer survival than the medians observed in ANLL patients who have no detectable abnormality. This discussion will emphasize certain specific aberrations that occur frequently and also appear to be of exceptional biological interest.

Chromosomal Gain and Loss

Although the karyotypes of patients with ANLL may be variable, both the nonrandom gain and loss of chromosomes and involvement in structural rearrangements are evident. Each of the autosomes and sex chromosomes have been observed to contribute to the numerical changes. Some chromosomes are clearly over-represented as gains or losses, while others are under-represented. Thus, a gain of chromosome 8, the most frequent abnormality seen in ANLL, occurs in approximately 13% of cases. Loss of chromosome 7, another frequent numerical change, occurs in 9% and loss of chromosome 5 in 6%. A gain of either of these chromosomes is rarely observed. It is interesting to note that gains or losses of the other autosomes seldom occur as the sole abnormality. Thus, these abnormalities likely represent secondary events occurring as a result of clonal evolution rather than primary chromosomal changes. Loss of the Y chromosome, the second most frequent numerical change in these patients, or loss of the X chromosome often occurs in association with an 8;21 translocation. Loss of a Y chromosome as the sole abnormality has been described, but the significance of this abnormality is uncertain because a missing Y chromosome has also been reported in bone marrow cells of hematologically normal males, particularly those over 60 years old. In contrast, the t(8;21) in acute myeloblastic leukemia (AML-M2) is usually observed in younger adults.

Specific Structural Rearrangements

The 8;21 translocation in acute myeloblastic leukemia (M2): In 1973, Rowley first described a balanced translocation between chromosomes 8 and 21 [t(8;21)(q22;q22)]. It is observed in approximately 10% of abnormal cases of ANLL. The t(8;21) has been found to be the most frequent abnormality in children with ANLL. This abnormality initially appeared to be restricted to patients with a diagnosis of M2 leukemia (acute myeloblastic leukemia with maturation) according to the FAB classification. However, several patients have had a diagnosis of acute myelomonocytic leukemia (M4).

Although the M2 type of ANLL is heterogeneous, the presence of the t(8;21) identifies a morphologically and clinically distinct subset. In this disorder, blasts tend to have indented nuclei, and the cytoplasm is generally basophilic with a prominent paranuclear hof that may contain a few azurophilic granules. Promyelocytes, myelocytes, and metamyelocytes are often quite prominent and may be large. Their cytoplasm has a waxy, orange appearance and lacks a granular texture in Romanowski-stained specimens. Auer rods are easily identified, and several may be seen in a single cell. Bone marrow eosinophilia is also common.

AML-M2 with the t(8;21) appears to have a favorable prognosis. The median age of these patients is approximately 25-30 years, significantly younger than that of patients with ANLL overall. The complete remission rate is uniformly high, and with intensive post-remission consolidation chemotherapy, the expected disease-free survival exceeds 2 years, after which time relapses are uncommon.

The 15;17 translocation in acute promyelocytic leukemia (M3): A structural rearrangement involving the long arms of chromosomes 15 and 17 in acute promyelocytic leukemia (APL-M3) was first recognized by Rowley and colleagues in 1977. For many years, the precise breakpoints involved in this translocation were controversial. The rearrangement was previously defined as t(15;17)(q22;q21), however, the break on chromosome 17 has recently been designated as q11-12 (Le Beau, unpublished data). The detection of this abnormality appears to depend upon the use of short-term bone marrow culture techniques. In our laboratory, each of 50 patients with APL whom we have examined have had a t(15;17). The microgranular variant of APL (M3V) also is characterized by the t(15;17). This rearrangement is highly specific for APL and has not been found in patients with any other type of leukemia or with a solid tumor.

Inv(16) and t(16;16) in acute myelomonocytic leukemia with abnormal eosinophils (M4Eo): Another recently identified clinical-cytogenetic association involves acute myelomonocytic leukemia with abnormal eosinophils (AMMoL-M4Eo). In 1983, Arthur and Bloomfield described five cases (three with AML-M2 and two with AMMoL-M4 leukemia) in which the bone marrow contained an excess of eosinophils (8-54%); all five patients were reported to have a deletion of chromosome 16 [del(16q)]. In the same year, Le Beau and colleagues initially reported on a related entity in 18 patients, all of whom had M4 leukemia with eosinophils that showed alterations of morphology, cytochemical reactions, and ultrastructure; these included the presence of large and irregular basophilic granules and positive reactions with periodic-acid-Schiff and chloroacetate esterase. Many of these patients did not have an increased percentage of marrow eosinophils; one-third had fewer than 5% eosinophils. Fifteen patients had a pericentric inversion of chromosome 16, inv(16)(p13q22), and in three patients a reciprocal translocation involving both chromosome 16 homologues [t(16;16)(p13;q22)] was noted. Among our M4 patients, 23% have had an inv(16) or t(16;16). Patients with inv(16) or t(16;16) have a good response to intensive chemotherapy. In our updated series, 25 (78%) of 32 treated patients entered a complete remission. The median survival for all 32 treated patients was longer than 66 weeks, and the median survival for those 25 patients who had a complete remission is longer than 104 weeks. This survival markedly exceeds the median of 29 weeks realized by 58 treated AMMoL patients who did not have this chromosomal rearrangement.

<u>Rearrangements of the long arm of chromosome 11 in acute monoblastic leukemia (M5)</u>: In 1980, Berger and co-workers first reported a higher than expected frequency of abnormalities of the long arm of chromosome 11 (11q) in patients with acute monocytic leukemia. In an expanded series of cases, rearrangements of 11q were observed in 35% of patients with M5, and the investigators emphasized an especially strong association between abnormalities of 11q and the poorly differentiated form of acute monoblastic leukemia (M5a). Rowley noted that the association between 11q abnormalities and M5a was particularly strong in children.

Several different rearrangements involving band 11q23 have been associated with ANLL. Most are translocations or deletions. The other chromosome involved in the translocations is variable but most frequently is chromosome 9 [t(9;11)(p22;q23)]. Less often chromosomes 10, 17, or 19 are involved: t(10;11)(p11-15;q23), t(11;17)(q23;q25), t(11;19)(q23;p13).

Although abnormalities of 11q are clearly correlated with M5, the association is not as strong as between the t(15;17) and M3. Abnormalities of 11q are seen in about 35% of all M5 patients and in slightly less than one half of the patients with M5a. Conversely, 11q abnormalities may be seen in ANLL other than M5 (most commonly M4), and some translocations involving 11q have been observed in patients with acute lymphoblastic leukemia (ALL).

Kaneko and associates recently reported on 11 patients who had hematologic malignancies associated with abnormalities of 11q23. Eight of the 11 were classified primarily on the basis of morphologic characteristics and cytochemical stains as having ALL or lymphoblastic lymphoma, including two of four patients with the t(9;11). These investigators theorized that acute leukemias associated with various abnormalities of 11q23 originate in a multipotential stem cell that is capable of differentiating along myeloid and/or lymphoid pathways. Another cytogenetic abnormality associated with a leukemia whose biologic features support this hypothesis is the t(4;11). Nevertheless, although acute leukemia associated with the t(11;19) has been reported both in patients with ANLL and in those with ALL, commitment to the lymphoid pathway has not been demonstrated either by immunologic marker studies or by the demonstration of clonal immunoglobulin or T-cell-receptor gene rearrangements in patients with the t(9;11), t(10;11), and t(11;17). To resolve this issue, it will be necessary to examine more cases using these techniques.

T(3;3) and inv(3) in ANLL with thrombocytosis: Rowley and colleagues initially reported on the presence of normal or elevated platelet counts in two patients with ANLL and structural abnormalities of the long arm of chromosome 3. These patients were found to have numerous micromegakaryocytes in their bone marrow. Additional patients who had identical or closely related cytogenetic abnormalities as well as thrombocytosis were subsequently reported by other investigators.

We recently studied 14 patients with abnormalities of 3q and ANLL or MDS, and confirmed an association of certain cytogenetic abnormalities with thrombocytosis in ANLL patients. The specific cytogenetic abnormalities associated with thrombocytosis in these patients involve bands 3q21 and 3q26 simultaneously, and they include the inv(3)(q21q26), t(3;3)(q21;q26), and the ins(5;3)(q14;q21q26). Seven of our eight patients with these abnormalities had platelet counts exceeding 100,000/microliter before the initiation of cytoreductive therapy. Four patients had significant thrombocytosis with platelet counts up to 1,731,000/microliter.

As might be expected, the most consistent bone marrow finding in these patients is an increase in the number of megakaryocytes, many of which are morphologically abnormal. In some of the patients, nearly all of the identifiable megakaryocytes are micromegakaryocytes. A few circulating megakaryoblasts were identified by the presence of platelet peroxidase activity in one of two patients whom we studied with this reaction. These histopathological findings are not indicative of acute megakaryoblastic leukemia.

The 6;9 translocation in ANLL with increased basophils: A translocation involving chromosomes 6 and 9 [t(6;9)(p23;q34)] was first described in two patients by Rowley and Potter in 1976 and later in 3 patients by Vermaelen and colleagues but no common features were detected. We have subsequently studied seven additional patients with this translocation. Patients with a t(6;9) comprise about 2% of our patients with ANLL. Eight of these nine patients had an increase in the number of basophils in the bone marrow ranging from 1.5 to 12%; the normal value is 0.2%. Because the marrow in all biopsy specimens was hypercellular, this represented a marked increase in the total basophil count. The basophils appeared to be morphologically normal. Only five of 163 ANLL patients whom we studied had increased numbers of marrow basophils (>1%) in the absence of the t(6;9). Of the nine t(6;9) patients, five were classified as AML-M2, three as AMMoL-M4, and one as AML-M1. The median age was 38 years, which is lower than that for ANLL patients overall. As a group, patients with a t(6;9) have responded poorly to intensive remission induction therapy. It is of interest that the breakpoint in chromosome 9 is in the same band as the break in the t(9;22) in CML and that a marked increase in basophils is a common feature of Ph^1+ CML. It is possible that, in both translocations, the break affects the function of a gene that is involved in the regulation of basophil proliferation and is located in this segment of 9q34. At the present time, there is no evidence for a break in the ABL gene, as described for the t(9;22).

THERAPY-RELATED MYELODYSPLASTIC SYNDROMES AND ACUTE NONLYMPHOCYTIC LEUKEMIA

Of increasing interest have been characteristic chromosomal abnormalities found in patients who develop a therapy-related MDS or ANLL (t-MDS or t-ANLL) after prior chemotherapy and/or radiation therapy for an earlier disorder, such as Hodgkin's disease, non-Hodgkin's lymphoma, carcinoma, rheumatoid arthritis, or renal transplantation. Two-thirds of these patients are first recognized by evidence of myelodysplasia, marrow failure, and pancytopenia. Not uncommonly, the initial malignant disease is still present at the time of the secondary bone marrow dysfunction. The interval between initial cytotoxic therapy and subsequent t-MDS/t-ANLL is about 5 years although the range is very broad (about 1-1/2 years - 18 years). Often, all 3 hematopoietic cell lines appear to be involved in the secondary malignancy. Precise subtyping by the FAB criteria used for ANLL de novo is seldom possible. Initially, the marrow may be hypocellular and fibrotic. Over time, myeloid blast cells accumulate in the marrow and blood. Half of patients diagnosed with t-MDS (<30% marrow blasts) will evolve to t-ANLL within a median of 6 months, but the other half will die of infectious or hemorrhagic complications of pancytopenia first.

In this section we will summarize the findings in our own series of 63 patients with t-MDS/t-ANLL. Twenty-three had Hodgkin's disease, 10 had non-Hodgkin's lymphoma (NHL), five had multiple myeloma, one had hairy cell leukemia, 21 had various solid tumors, and three had had a renal transplant. Thirty-one of the patients had received both radiotherapy and chemotherapy prior to the development of their second malignancy, and 21 patients had only chemotherapy. Eleven patients had only radiotherapy and, in 9 of these, major areas containing active marrow had been irradiated. The median time between the original diagnosis and the diagnosis of secondary bone marrow dysfunction was 56 months and did not vary significantly depending on the primary disorder or the primary treatment.

In contrast to our concurrent series of patients with ANLL de novo in which 54% of patients had clonal chromosomal abnormalities, 61 of 63 (97%) patients with therapy-related malignancies were chromosomally abnormal. More importantly, one or both of two consistent changes were noted in 55 of the 61 (90%) patients with abnormalities. Fourteen patients had loss of one chromosome 5 (six patients) or an interstitial deletion of the q arm [del(5q)] (eight patients), and 24 patients had loss of one chromosome 7 (22 patients) or a del(7q) (two patients). An additional 17 patients had abnormalities of both chromosomes 5 and 7. A comparison of the frequency of abnormalities for each chromosome in de novo ANLL and t-ANLL revealed that chromosomes 5 and 7 as well as chromosomes 1, 4, 12, 14 and 18 were involved significantly more frequently in the latter group of patients. Of the six patients with abnormalities involving chromosomes other than 5 and/or 7, it is noteworthy that two patients had a gain of chromosome 8 as their sole abnormality, and both patients with secondary APL had the t(15;17)(q22;q11-12).

Chromosomal abnormalities are found in most patients with t-MDS prior to the evolution of overt leukemia, and these changes are often multiple and complex. Aberrations involving chromosomes 5 or 7 either alone or in combination with other changes again account for the majority of cytogenetic abnormalities in t-MDS. In the University of Chicago series, 97% of 48 patients with t-MDS demonstrated a clonal chromosomal abnormality, and 87% had abnormalities of chromosomes No. 5 and/or 7. Thus, the detection of a clonal abnormality in a pancytopenic patient is convincing evidence of the existence of a malignant secondary neoplasm even though the percentage of blasts in the marrow is not yet elevated.

The high frequency of abnormalities of chromosomes 5 and 7 in patients who have t-MDS/t-ANLL led investigators to hypothesize that abnormalities of these chromosomes are the hallmark of mutagen-induced myeloid leukemias. Further support for this hypothesis was provided by several studies which demonstrated a higher frequency of abnormalities of chromosomes 5 and/or 7 in the malignant cells of ANLL patients who have a history of occupational exposure to potential mutagens than in those patients who have no such exposure history.

The variability in the chromosomal breakpoints observed in the deletions of 5q and 7q in primary and therapy-related MDS or ANLL suggests that the juxtaposition of identical gene sequences, an event that may occur as a result of rearrangements such as translocations, is not a likely mechanism in these secondary disorders. Rather, the relevant genetic event may be the loss of critical genes as a result of the loss of a whole chromosome or a deletion, thereby allowing the expression of a mutant allele on the remaining chromosome, or resulting in the homozygous inactivation of a leukemia "suppressor" gene, a mechanism that has recently been demonstrated for the pathogenesis of retinoblastoma, another human tumor that is frequently associated with loss or deletion of a chromosome (No. 13).

By cytogenetic analysis of the deletions of 5q, we previously identified a region (termed the critical region), consisting of bands 5q23 and q31, that was deleted in all patients. It is now known that this DNA region contains the genes for several hematopoietic growth factors, namely, GM-CSF (granulocyte-macrophage colony-stimulating factor) and interleukin-3 (multi-CSF), and is flanked by the genes for CSF-1 (macrophage-CSF) and FMS (CSF-1 receptor). Other genes that have recently been mapped to the critical region include the gene encoding CD14, a myeloid-specific differentiation-associated antigen, and the EGR1 gene, which encodes a DNA-binding protein. The latter gene is of particular interest because other DNA-binding proteins have proven to play important roles in the regulation of gene expression. The transforming sequence MET is located at 7q22-31, near the consistently deleted segment of this chromosome. Neutrophil chemotactic factor is encoded by a gene on chromosome 7, and this activity may be deficient in patients with monosomy 7.

REFERENCES

Bitter MA, Le Beau MM, Rowley JD, Larson RA, Golomb HM, Vardiman JW (1987) Associations between morphology, karyotype, and clinical features in myeloid leukemias. Human Path 18:211-225

Bloomfield CD, Trent JM, van den Berghe H (1987) Report of the committee on structural chromosome changes in neoplasia (Human Gene Mapping 9). Cytogenet Cell Genet 46:344-366

Le Beau MM, Larson RA (1988) Hematologic malignancies. In: King RA, Rotter JJ, Motulsky AG (eds) The Genetic Basis of Common Diseases. Oxford University Press, New York, in press

Mitelman F (1988) Catalog of Chromosome Aberrations in Cancer (3rd edition). Alan R. Liss, New York, p 1

Rowley JD (1984) Biological implications of consistent chromosome rearrangements in leukemia and lymphoma. Cancer Res 44:3159-3165

Second MIC Cooperative Study Group (1988) Morphologic, immunologic and cytogenetic (MIC) working classification of the acute myeloid leukaemias. Br J Haematol 68:487-494

Radiation Induced Deletion of Chromosome 2 in Myeloid Leukemogenesis

Nechama Haran-Ghera

Department of Chemical Immunology, The Weizmann Institute of Science, Rehovot 76100, Israel

RADIATION MYELOID LEUKEMOGENESIS IN THE MOUSE

The majority of experimental radiation leukemia studies have been concerned with thymic lymphomas whereas only a few have been reported on radiation induced myeloid leukemia. The early systematic studies involved myeloid leukemia induction in the RF strain by exposure to whole body ionizing radiation. This strain was shown to be susceptible to both radiation induced lymphoid and myeloid leukemia (Upton et al., 1958). The susceptibility to myeloid leukemia induction by X-rays increased progressively during the first month of life and did not decrease with advancing age, contrary to reduced susceptibility to lymphoma induction with age increase. For the induction of myeloid leukemia there appeared to be an effective threshold dose in the neighborhood of 150-300r, causing 30-40% tumor development. The incidence of myeloid leukemia was not affected by fractionation of the radiation dose in contrast to thymic lymphoma incidence being increased by fractionated irradiation. Partial body irradiation (300r) of the upper body (shielding the pelvis and lower extremities) reduced leukemia incidence (11% versus 38% in whole body exposed RF mice) (Upton et al., 1958; Upton et al., 1966). Males were found to be more susceptible to radiation induced myeloid leukemia than females (females being more susceptible to radiation induced thymic lymphomas). Ovariectomy did not significantly affect the incidence of myeloid leukemia in females nor did orchidectomy alter significantly the rate of myeloid leukemia induction in males (Upton et al., 1958). Thymectomy had no effect on myeloid leukemogenesis whereas splenectomy had an inhibitory action on the induction rate (13% versus 35% in intact RF mice exposed to 300r). Splenectomy even as late as 1 month after irradiation afforded inhibition. The spleen was actually shown to be the major site of neoplastic infiltration in myeloid leukemia development and might thus play an important role in the pathogenesis of the disease. It is noteworthy that removal of the spleen had no significant effect on the induction of lymphoma. Specific pathogen free RF mice were shown to be less susceptible to radiation induced myeloid leukemia than the conventionally reared counterparts (Upton et al., 1966). These observations on myeloid pathogenesis might indicate that a complex interaction among host factors and extrenuous agents affect the development of the disease.

A limited number of mice strains were actually found to be moderatly susceptible to myeloid leukemia development (20-30%) following the optimum X-ray dose, a single exposure to 150-350r, at a mean latency period of one year. Among these strains are the SJL/J (Haran-Ghera et al., 1967), CBA/H (Major and Mole, 1978) and C3H/H (Hirashima et al., 1983) mice. In SJL/J mice myeloid leukemia induction was also observed following repeated feedings with 7,12-dimethylbenz(a) anthracene (DMBA), inducing 27% myeloid leukemia at a mean age of 180 days (Haran-Ghera et, 1967). Comparative studies on radiation induced leukemias in CBA/H mice suggested differences in the mechanism of radiation induced myeloid and lymphoid leukemia (Mole, 1986). In radiation induced myeloid leukemia a progressive reduction in frequency of the disease from 24% to 6.6% was observed when the time interval between two equal exposures was increased to 3-7 days. Thus, the leukemia inducing effect of the first exposure (125r) interacting with the corresponding effect produced by the second same dose declined with time (3-7 days). It was suggested that the radiation induced initiation effect is not an

Current Topics in Microbiology and Immunology, Vol. 149

immediate permanent change but requires to be "fixed" in some way. The injection of normal syngeneic bone marrow cells (3 x 10^7 cells) only at an appropriate and narrowly defined time (3 days after irradiation) accelerated development of myeloid leukemia (Mole, 1986). These results suggest that after the inductive effect of radiation, additional factors could modify the latency and incidence of myeloid leukemia.

COLEUKEMOGENIC EFFECTS OF CORTICOSTEROIDS

Cortisone administered to RF mice after irradiation was shown to inhibit lymphoma development but was without effect on the induction of myeloid leukemia (Upton and Furth, 1954). Enhancement of X-ray induced myeloid leukemia in C3H male mice was attempted by additional treatment with prednisone and/or metyrapone without much success ((Hayata et al., 1983) and personal communication by Dr. M. Seki). In order to test if adrenal steroid imbalance could affect the incidence of radiation-induced myeloid leukemia in SJL/J mice, we tested the coleukemogenic effect of hydrocortisone acetate, prednisone, metyrapone and ACTH as coleukemogenic agents to the initial radiation (Resnitzky et al., 1985). Exposure of female SJL/J mice to 300r whole body irradiation induced about 20% acute myeloid leukemia (AML) at a mean latency of 300 days. Additional treatment of intact mice with corticosteroids before and/or after irradiation increased tumor incidence to 40-50% and to a higher incidence (75%) in thymectomized mice treated with prednisone. Negative feedback on the T cell level introduced by thymectomy and corticosteroid treatment, thereby eliminating some T cell populations, may favor the proliferation of myeloid precursors. An increase in AML incidence (50%) was also observed when metyrapone was administered after X-ray treatment. In contrast, no coleukemogenic effect to radiation was observed when mice were treated with ACTH. The efficient coleukemogenic effect of steroids, when their administration was delayed after irradiation, suggested that radiation may contribute to the induction of AML initiation and the additional millieu of hormonal imbalance could further trigger the proliferation of the immortalized transformed cells.

It is interesting to stress that only myeloid type of acute leukemia appeared in all the radiation-coleukemogenic combinations tested. The myeloid nature of the leukemic cells infiltrating the different organs was established by typical morphological and cytochemical findings for granulocytic differentiation (Resnitzky et al., 1985). Interestingly, also exclusively AML is the type of the secondary leukemia arising increasingly in cancer patients treated previously with alkylating agents, irradiation, steroids and other cytotoxic drugs (Pedersen-Bjergaard and Olesen-Larsen, 1982; Brenner et al., 1984; Pedersen-Bjergaard et al., 1984; De Vita et al., 1970). In accordance with these findings we recently tested the coleukemogenic effect of repeated treatments of prednisone and cytophosphane (five alternative weekly treatments, the whole treatment lasting 10 weeks after exposure to 300r). This combined coleukemogenic treatment following radiation increased AML incidence to 92% at a mean latency of 265 days. One single prednisone injection after radiation or five repeated injections yielded a similar 50% AML incidence; five repeated treatments with cytophosphane following 300r did not increase AML incidence beyond the radiation induced AML incidence; both agents without initial exposure to radiation had no leukemogenic effect (Haran-Ghera et al., in press). Thus, the combined coleukemogenic treatment seemed to promote the proliferation and progression of the radiation induced preleukemic clone to overt AML.

CHROMOSOME ANALYSIS OF RADIATION INDUCED MYELOID LEUKEMIA

Radiation induced myeloid leukemia in several mouse strains was found to be associated with abnormalities of chromosome (ch) 2. Consistent occurrence of partial deletion of ch 2 in myeloid leukemia of irradiated C3H/He and RFM mice was described by Hayata and colleagues several years ago (Hayata et al., 1983). Among 52 radiation induced myeloid leukemia analyzed, 49 tumors had the characteristic ch 2 deletion, in about 30% of the tested tumors an anomaly in ch 6 was observed and anomalies of ch 3 and 9 were the next most frequent, appearing in 14 cases each. Loss of the Y chromosome was also observed in 34 out of 46 male AML cases. Seven different types of deletions, varying in size and in their mode of formation, were observed among the karyotyped tumors classified as myeloblastic leukemias, granulocytic leukemias, myelomonocytic leukemias and monocyte leukemias. One common missing segment between regions 2C and 2D was observed in the deleted ch 2 among the different tumors tested. These results suggest that murine radiation induced myeloid leukemia is influenced by genetic information on ch 2 within regions C and D. Karyotype analysis of radiation induced myeloid leukemias of CBA/H mice showed consistent chromosomal changes in about 90% of AML (15/16) involving deletion and/or translocation of ch 2. Abnormalities of ch 2 were centered on an interstitial region with most breakpoints in the C2 and/or E5 G bands (Silver et al., 1987). Of the 15 ch 2 events scored, 8 were deletions (predominantly interstitial) and 7 were translocations (often incomplete), involving exchange between the two ch 2 homologues (3/7) or between ch 2 with other chromosomes. Thus, the C2-E5 region of chromosome 2 might encode gene(s) that are involved in AML development. Azumi and Sachs (1977) described chromosome mapping of 10 clones of myeloid leukemia cells. Six clones derived from radiation induced AML in SJL/J mice showed a loss of a piece of one chromosome 2. The size of the missing piece varied in the six clones from a smaller to a larger piece. There were in some clones other abnormalities including trisomy of ch 12 and 15. The other four clones, isolated from a myeloid leukemia cell line in culture obtained from a spontaneous myeloid leukemia in a female SL mouse had a normal diploid karyotype. Recently, cytogenetic analysis of AML induced in SJL/J mice by radiation with or without further corticosteroid treatment was carried out in our laboratory (Trakhtenbrot et al., 1988). Cells from eight AMLs induced by exposure to 300r only and 12 AMLs induced by radiation and additional corticosteroid treatment were karyotyped. The control group included two age groups: ten female mice aged 9 months that looked grossly normal (and confirmed histologically) and eight females aged 14 months, five of them developed spontaneously reticulum cell neoplasms reclassified recently as B cell neoplasia that is characteristic to this strain (Wanebo et al., 1966; Pattengale and Firth, 1983). All tested AMLs had a common characteristic deletion of one ch 2. The shortened latency and increased incidence in AML development due to the coleukemogenic treatment did not affect the ch 2 deletion tumor pattern. Other chromosome rearrangements were observed in some tumors with a different pattern for each tumor, probably occurring during tumor progression. Analysis of bone marrow and spleen cells from untreated SJL/J mice from both age groups revealed that all mice had a normal karyotype, irrespective to the presence of spontaneous neoplasms observed in the older tested mice. Thus, the absence of ch 2 deletion in animals with spontaneous B neoplasms may suggest that these tumors and the radiation induced AML in SJL/J mice involve two different target cells. The deletion in ch 2 varied in size and its manner of formation, but each tumor had only one characteristic type of deletion in all cells involved. According to the morphological patterns, the deleted ch 2 could be classified into 5 types in relation with the missing region or interstitial deletion. The common missing part in all 5 types of ch 2 deletion involved segment D through G. This common deleted area matches with the missing segment between regions C and D described in Hayata's studies (1983). Thus, the loss of the genetic information in this similar region in different strains of mice developing radiation induced myeloid leukemia may be responsible for the generation of the disease by radiation. It is interesting to point out that the spontaneous occurring myeloid leukemia in the SL mouse (Azumi and Sachs, 1977) and karyotype analysis of 3 spontaneous occurring myeloid tumors in thymectomized AKR mice (unpublished data) showed a normal diploid karyotype.

The role of gene deletion as a predisposition in tumorigenesis has been extensively studied in connection with retinoblastoma and neuroblastoma (Yunis and Ransey, 1978; Yunis, 1983). Deletion of the long arm of ch 5 ($5q^-$) often together with deletion of ch 7 was described in human secondary non-lymphocytic (ANLL) leukemia (Rowley et al., 1981; Le Beau et al., 1986). The oncogene c-fms that encodes for CSF-1 was recently assigned to human ch 5 (Groffen et al., 1983; Roussel et al., 1983). The gene for GM-CSF, also located on ch 5 has been recently shown to be deleted in patients with myeloidysplastic syndrome and in acute non-lymphocyte leukemia (Le Beau et al., 1986). It has been suggested that loss or inactivation of negative regulatory genes through deletions may affect tumor development by derepressing other critical genes (Kundson, 1985; Atkin, 1985).

The c-abl gene that has been implicated in the pathogenesis of human CML (Nowell and Croce, 1986) was mapped by Goff et al. (1982) to the mouse chromosome 2. A possible correlation between the localization of c-abl and the breakpoint in the deletion implicated in radiation induced AML seemed worthwhile testing. A brief recent report involving studies on radiation induced AML in CBA/H mice (Silver et al., 1988) suggests that the proto-oncogene c-abl is actually not involved in the ch 2 rearrangement that characterizes murine myeloid leukemia. It would of course be interesting to investigate the possible role of other oncogenes related with hematopoietic proliferation, differentiation and maturation in the genesis of murine radiation induced AML.

DELETION OF CH 2 IS AN EARLY EVENT IN AML DEVELOPMENT

Since all AMLs induced in SJL/J mice by exposure to radiation with or without further coleukemogenic treatment were characterized by a deletion of one ch 2, the deletion seems to be a necessary step in the radiation induced tumorigenic process. Our working hypothesis was that deletion of ch 2 may contribute to the initial radiation induced transformation and other additional host factors could further affect the pattern of differentiation and proliferation of the transformed cells. It seemed therefore of interest to test the possible occurrence of the deletion among bone marrow cells following exposure to radiation, long before overt leukemia is observed. Female SJL/J mice were exposed to 300r whole body irradiation and 4 months later (when the mice looked grossly normal) the occurrence of cells expressing deletion of ch 2 among their marrow cells was tested. About 80% (14/17) of the mice tested had different levels of cells with deletion 2. In mice diagnosed grossly and histologically as normal, the average deletion incidence was 10-15%, versus 30-60% in mice that looked grossly normal but following histological examination they were diagnosed as preleukemic (due to sporadic leukemic foci observed in their spleens) (Trakhtenbrot et al., 1988). Usually one type of deletion was found in all the cells involved in the individual mouse tested. But in several cases two or three different types of deletions were observed, probably representing initial polyclonal transformation. In the final AML one type of ch 2 deletion in 100% of the leukemic cells was observed, thereby suggesting the derivation of the tumor from a single altered cell. Analysis of bone marrow from mice tested 4 months after exposure to 300r plus one single injection of dexamethasone revealed cells with ch 2 deletion in all treated mice (12/12). The percentage of cells with deletion 2 among the karyotyped cells (50-70 cells) was higher (20-30%) than in mice exposed to 300r only (10-15%) (unpublished results). A certain threshold level of cells with deletion 2, beyond 20%, seems to be essential for the actual overt AML development. In mice tested 4 months after 300r, 28% of mice had more than 20% deleted cells among the marrow karyotyped cells versus 60% with the additional Dexamethasone-coleukemogenic treatment. These deleted cell levels in the two different treatment modalities match with the final AML incidence observed following these two types of leukemogenic treatment (Resnitzky et al., 1985).

To ascertain that bone marrow from mice 4 months after leukemogenic treatment does indeed contain cells that have the potential to develop into AML (preleukemic cells) some transplantation studies were carried out. Bone marrow cells removed from normal or irradiated (300r) plus Dexamethrasone (0.5 mg subc.) treated mice were injected i.v. into SJL/J recipient mice that received 500r whole body irradiation 1-3 hr before cell injection. Transfer of normal bone marrow (matching age to the treated donor mice) resulted in 85% development of the spontaneous B cell neoplasia characteristic to SJL/J mice (Wanebo et al., 1966). In contrast, the irradiated bone marrow ((4×10^7 cells) induced 75% AML at a mean latent period of 120 days (unpublished results). Similar AML induction was also obtained following transfer of spleen cells taken from the same treated donors. Thus, several months following the leukemogenic treatment (that eventually induces 50-70% AML following exposure to 300r + Dexamethasone) the treated mice carry preleukemic cells, probably involving the deleted ch 2 clones. In some preliminary studies, in an attempt to define the subpopulation that contains the preleukemic cells, we separated the marrow on the basis of cell size and density (by counterflow centrifugal elutriation). The preliminary results suggest that the bone marrow fraction mostly enriched in CFU-s yields a high AML incidence (80-100%) following transfer into the compatible recipients.

Our findings revealing the ch 2 deletion in the preleukemic phase suggest that the deletion is an early event in tumor formation, and not related to tumor progression. Although the radiation induced AML incidence after an average latent period of 300 days ranges only between 20-30% (Resnitzky et al., 1985; Trakhtenbrot et al., 1988) we have demonstrated that 80%-100% of the irradiated mice carried cells with ch 2 deletion among their marrow population 120 days after the exposure. This discrepancy between the presence of deleted preleukemic clones and overt leukemia incidence clearly indicates that ch 2 deletion is an essential factor and an early event in AML formation, but is not always sufficient to cause malignancy. Additional coleukemogenic treatments, like corticoids used in our studies, are required for the promotion of the radiation initiated clones, yielding ultimately a high AML incidence.

ACKNOWLEDGMENT

This work was supported by a grant from the Ebner Family Leukemia Research Foundation at the Weizmann Institute of Science, in Memory of Alfred Ebner.

REFERENCES

Atkin NB (1985) Antioncogenes. Lancet 11: 1189-1190.

Azumi JI, Sachs L (1977) Chromosome mapping of the genes that control differentiation and malignancy in myeloid leukemic cells. Proc Natl Acad Sci USA 74: 253-257.

Brenner B, Carter A, Sharon R, Tatarsky I (1984) Acute leukemia following chemotherapy and radiation therapy. A report of 15 cases. Oncology 41: 83-87.

De Vita V, Serpick A, Carbone P (1970) Combination chemotherapy in the treatment of advanced Hodgkin's disease. Ann Intern Med 73: 881-885.

Goff SP, D'Eustachio P, Ruddle F.H., Baltimore D (1982). Chromosomal assignment of endogenous proto-oncogene c-abl. Science 218: 1317-1319.

Groffen J, Heisterkamp N, Spun M et al. (1983) Chromosomal localization of the human c-fms oncogene. Nucleic Acid Res 11: 6331-6339.

Haran-Ghera N, Kotler M, Meshorer A (1967) Studies on leukemia development in the SJL/J strain of mice. J Natl Cancer Inst 39: 653-661.

Haran-Ghera N, Trakhtenbrot L, Resnitzky P, Peled A. Preleukemia in experimental leukemogenesis. Leukemia, in press.

Hayata I, Seki M, Yoshida K et al. (1983) Chromosomal aberrations observed in 52 mouse myeloid leukemias. Cancer Res 43: 367-373.

Hirashima K, Basho M, Hayata I et al. (1983) Experimental study on the mechanism of radiation induced myeloid leukemogenesis. Expt Hemato 11 (Suppl. 14) 157-164.

Knudson AG (1985) Hereditary cancer, oncogenes and antioncogenes. Cancer Res 45: 1437-1443.

Le Beau MM, Albain KS, Larson RA et al. (1986) Clinical and cytogenetic correlation in 63 patients with therapy-related myelodysplastic syndromes and acute non-lymphocytic leukemia: Further evidence for characteristic abnormalities of chromosome 5 and 7. J Clin Oncol 4: 325-332.

Le Beau MM, Westbrook CA, Diaz MO et al. (1986) Evidence for the involvement of GM-CSF and FMS in the deletion ($5q^-$) in myeloid disorders. Science 231: 984-987.

Major IR, Mole RH (1978) Myeloid leukemia in X-ray irradiated CBA mice. Nature 272: 455-456.

Mole RH (1986) Radiation-induced acute myeloid leukemia in the mouse: experimental observations in vivo with implications for hypotheses about the basis of carcinogenesis. Leuk Res 10: 859-865.

Nowell PC, Croce M (1986) Chromosomes, genes and cancer. Am J Pathol 125: 8-15, 1986.

Pattengale, PK, Firth Ch.H (1983) Immunomorphologic classification of spontaneous lymphoid cell neoplasms occurring in female BALB/c mice. J Natl Cancer Inst 70: 169-179.

Pedersen-Bjergaard J, Olesen-Larsen S (1982) Incidence of acute nonlymphocytic leukemia, preleukemia and acute myeloproliferative syndrome up to 10 years after treatment of Hodgkin's disease. New England J Med 307: 965-971.

Pedersen-Bjergaard J, Philip P, Tingaard-Petersen N. et al. (1984) Acute nonlymphocytic leukemia, preleukemia and acute myeloproliferative syndrome secondary to treatment of other malignant diseases. Cancer 54: 452-459.

Resnitzky P, Esterov Z, Haran-Ghera N (1985) High incidence of acute myeloid leukemia in SJL/J mice after X-irradiation and corticosteroids. Leuk Res 9: 1519-1528.

Roussel MF, Sherr Ch.J, Barker P, Ruddle FH (1983) Molecular cloning of the c-fms locus and its assignment to human chromosomes. J Virol 48: 770-773.

Rowely J, Golomb HM, Varaliman JW (1981) Non random chromosome abnormalities in acute leukemia and dysmyelopoietic syndromes in patients with previously treated malignant disease. Blood 58: 759-767.

Silver A, Breckon G, Masson WK, Malowany D, Cox R (1987) Studies on radiation myeloid leukemogenesis in the mouse. Radiation Research: Proceedings of the 8th Int. Congress of Radiation Res. vol. 2, ed. E.M. Filden, J.F. Fowler, J.H. Hendry and D. Scott (London: Taylor and Frances) p 494-500, 1987.

Silver A, Masson ARJ, Breckon WK, Cox R (1988) Preliminary molecular studies on two chromosome 2 encoded genes, c-abl and β2M, in radiation-induced murine myeloid leukaemias. Int J Radiat Biol 53: 57-63.

Trakhtenbrot L, Krauthgamer R, Resnitzky P., Haran-Ghera N (1988) Deletion of chromosome 2 is an early event in the development of radiation induced myeloid leukemia in SJL/J mice. Leukemia 2: 545-550.

Upton AC, Furth J (1954) The effect of cortisone on the development of spontaneous leukemia in mice and on its induction by irradiation. Blood 9: 686-695, 1954.

Upton AC, Wolff FF, Furth J, Kimball AW (1958) A comparison of the induction of myeloid and lymphoid leukemias in X-radiated RF mice. Cancer Res 18: 842-848.

Upton AC, Jenkins VK, Walburg HE, Tyndall RL, Conklin JW, Wald N (1966) Observations on viral, chemical and radiation-induced myeloid and lymphoid leukemias in RF mice. Natl Cancer Inst Monograph 22: 329-347.

Yunis J, Ransey M (1978) Retinoblastoma and sub-band deletion of chromosome 13. Am J Dis Child 132: 161-170.

Yunis J (1983) The chromosomal basis of human neoplasia. Science 221: 227-236.

Wanebo, HJ, Gallmeier WM, Boyse EA, Old L (1966) Paraproteinemia and reticulum cell sarcoma in an inbred mouse strain. Science 154: 901-903.

III. Disruption of "Oncogenes" by Virus Insertion in Murine Myeloid Tumorigenesis

Recombinant Inbred Mouse Strains: Models for Studying the Molecular Genetic Basis of Myeloid Tumorigenesis

Neal G. Copeland, Arthur M. Buchberg, Debra J. Gilbert and Nancy A. Jenkins

Mammalian Genetics Laboratory, BRI-Basic Research Program, NCI-Frederick Cancer Research Facility, Frederick, MD 21701

INTRODUCTION

Several inbred mouse strains have been derived that have a high spontaneous incidence of hematopoietic disease (reviewed by Gross 1983). Invariably, the high tumor incidence in these strains is causally associated with the expression of murine leukemia viruses (MuLV). Viruses expressed by these strains are inherited vertically, as normal Mendelian genes, or horizontally via infection of newborns through the mothers milk or of embryos, *in utero*. These viruses do not transform cells in culture and they do not carry oncogenes. They induce disease only after long latency periods, apparently by insertional activation of cellular genes (reviewed by Nusse, 1986).

Several known cellular genes have been shown to be activated by viral integration in murine hematopoietic tumors (Table 1). These genes include protooncogenes and genes encoding growth factors or growth factor receptors (Table 1). The mode of gene activation by viral integration in tumors is diverse (reviewed by Nusse 1986). Transcriptional promoters present in the viral long terminal repeat (LTR) can directly promote transcription of a nearby gene. Viruses can also activate gene expression by 1) an enhancement mechanism, 2) by integrating into an intron and thereby disrupting the protein coding domain, or 3) by integrating into 3' untranslated sequences. In the third case, gene expression may be enhanced by mRNA stabilization.

Conversely, the genes activated by viral integration in tumors may represent novel cellular genes involved in tumorigenesis. The somatically acquired proviruses in tumors serve as useful retrotransposon "tags" for the molecular identification of cellular loci involved in the disease process. In practice, these loci are identified by cloning proviral DNA-host cellular DNA junction fragments from virally induced tumors. Unique sequence cellular DNA probes flanking these proviruses are then identified and used to screen other tumors by Southern blot analysis to determine whether proviruses are integrated into the same regions in other tumors. Since retroviruses can integrate into many sites in the host genome, the detection of rearrangements at the same locus in several independent tumors suggests that the locus encodes a gene whose activation by viral integration predisposes cells to tumorigenesis. These loci have been termed common sites of viral integration.

Many common sites of viral integration have been identified in murine hematopoietic tumors (Table 2). The *Fim-2* common viral integration site identified in Friend MuLV (F-MuLV)-induced myeloblastic leukemias encodes the receptor for the hematopoietic growth factor, monocyte-macrophage colony-stimulating factor (M-CSF or CSF-1) (Gisselbrecht *et al.*, 1987). This growth factor receptor is a transmembrane protein with tyrosine kinase activity. The *Pim-1* common viral integration site identified in mink cell focus-forming

Current Topics in Microbiology and Immunology, Vol. 149

Table 1. Cellular genes activated by MuLV integration in murine hematopoietic tumors.

Gene Family	Locus Activated	Reference
Protooncogene	***Myc***	Corcoran ***et al.***, 1984 Selten ***et al.***, 1984 Li ***et al.***, 1984 Reicin ***et al.***, 1986 Wirchubsky ***et al.***, 1986 Mucenski ***et al.***, 1987a Warren ***et al.***, 1987
	Myb	Mushinski ***et al.***, 1983 Shen-Ong ***et al.***, 1984 Shen-Ong ***et al.***, 1986 Weinstein ***et al.***, 1986
	Kras	George ***et al.***, 1986
Growth Factor	***Csfm***	Baumbach, Stanley and Cole, 1987
Growth Factor Receptor	***Fms***	Gisselbrecht ***et al.***, 1987

(MCF) MuLV-induced T-cell lymphomas shows extensive homology with serine protein kinases (Selten ***et al.***, 1986). Activation of the ***Pim-1*** locus has also been reported to occur in B-cell lymphomas (Mucenski ***et al.***, 1987a; Hanecak ***et al.***, 1988). The ***Lck*** common viral integration site identified in a Moloney MuLV (Mo-MuLV)-induced T-cell lymphoma line encodes a novel cellular tyrosine protein kinase related to the ***Src*** protooncogene (Marth ***et al.*** 1985; Voronova and Sefton, 1986). These genes all demonstrate functional hallmarks expected for genes causally-associated with neoplastic disease. The results of these studies provide support for the utility of this approach for isolating novel genes involved in neoplastic disease.

RECOMBINANT INBRED MOUSE STRAINS

In addition to inbred strains, several recombinant inbred (RI) mouse strains have been developed for studying the molecular genetic basis of hematopoietic disease. RI strains are derived by systematic inbreeding following the cross of two inbred mouse strains (Taylor 1978). RI strains represent stable segregant populations resulting from the chance reassortment of the two parental genotypes. RI strains can be typed for any genes in which the two parental strains differ (protein polymorphism, restriction fragment length polymorphism, etc.), making them extremely useful for gene mapping experiments. RI strains derived from mice that differ in disease incidence provide unique resources for identifying and studying genes that affect the disease process. If the disease is virally-induced, the viruses also serve as useful retrotransposon tags for identifying cellular genes involved in the disease process in these RI strains. Because RI strains are inbred, all data are cumulative,

Table 2. Common Sites of Viral Integration in Murine Hematopoietic Tumors

Locus	Disease	Reference
Pim-1	T-cell lymphoma B-cell lymphoma	Cuypers *et al.*, 1984 Selten *et al.*, 1985 Wirschubsky *et al.*, 1986 Warren *et al.*, 1986 Mucenski *et al.*, 1987a Hanecak, Pattengale and Fan, 1988
Pim-2	T-cell lymphoma	Berns *et al.*, personal communication
Pvt-1	T-cell lymphoma	Graham, Adams and Cory, 1985 Mucenski *et al.*, 1987a
Fis-1	T-cell lymphoma Myeloid leukemia	Silver and Kozak, 1986 Mucenski *et al.*, 1987a
Lck	T-cell lymphoma	Marth *et al.*, 1985 Voronova and Sefton, 1986
Gin-1	T-cell lymphoma	Villemur *et al.*, 1987
Mlvi-1	T-cell lymphoma	Wirschubsky *et al.*, 1986 Mucenski *et al.*, 1987a
Mlvi-2	T-cell lymphoma	Mucenski *et al.*, 1987a
Fim-1	Myeloblastic leukemia	Sola *et al.*, 1986
Fim-2	Myeloblastic leukemia	Sola *et al.*, 1986 Gisselbrecht *et al.*, 1987
Fim-3	Myeloblastic leukemia	Bordereaux *et al.*, 1987
Evi-1	Myeloid leukemia	Mucenski *et al.*, 1988b
Evi-2	Myeloid leukemia	Buchberg *et al.*, 1988, unpublished results
Spi-1	Erythroleukemia	Moreau-Gachelin, Tavitian and Tambourin, 1988

and as new genes are identified, their effect, if any, on the disease process can be identified.

AKXD RI MOUSE STRAINS

The AKXD RI strains represent a valuable RI strain family for identifying and studying genes that affect susceptibility to lymphomas. These strains were derived by crossing mice from two inbred strains that differed significantly in lymphoma incidence, AKR/J and DBA/2J. AKR/J is the prototypic highly lymphomatous mouse strain; nearly all of these mice develop T-cell lymphomas by 7 to 16 months of age. The lymphoma incidence in DBA/2J mice is low.

The high incidence of lymphomas in AKR/J mice is associated with the expression of two endogenous ecotropic MuLV loci ***Emv-11*** and ***Emv-14*** (Jenkins ***et al.***, 1982a). MCF viruses have also been identified in both preleukemic and leukemic thymuses of AKR/J mice (Hartley ***et al.***, 1977; Herr and Gilbert, 1983; 1984). MCF viruses are not encoded directly in the AKR/J germline but are generated by multiple recombination events involving an ecotropic virus and at least two nonecotropic viruses (Quint ***et al.***, 1984). Whereas the ecotropic viruses are weakly leukemogenic, MCF viruses are highly leukemogenic when injected into susceptible hosts (Holland ***et al.***, 1985), suggesting that generation of MCF viruses is an important event in the development of T-cell lymphomas in AKR/J mice. Although DBA/2J mice also carry an endogenous ecotropic provirus, ***Emv-3***, this provirus carries a small mutation in the ***gag*** gene that inhibits its expression (Copeland ***et al.***, 1988). The low level of virus expression in DBA/2J mice is likely to be an important factor contributing to the low tumor incidence in this strain.

Lymphoma Susceptibility and Disease Type of 23 AKXD RI Strains

Among 23 AKXD RI strains analyzed for their tumor incidence, 21 strains developed tumors at high frequency (Mucenski ***et al.***, 1986; Gilbert, Taylor, Jenkins and Copeland, unpublished results). The average age of onset of tumors varied considerably among the different AKXD strains, suggesting that several loci affecting lymphoma susceptibility have segregated in these RI strains. The two AKXD strains with low tumor incidence did not inherit either highly expressed endogenous ecotropic proviral loci, ***Emv-11*** or ***Emv-14***, from the AKR/J parent, which likely accounts for their low susceptibility to tumors. Unexpectedly, only five strains were identified that developed primarily T-cell lymphomas like the parental AKR/J strain (Table 3). Five strains developed primarily B-cell lymphomas and one strain developed primarily myeloid tumors. Ten strains were susceptible to both T-cell and B-cell lymphomas. Thus, the AKXD strains have segregated for genes that not only affect lymphoma susceptibility but lymphoma type.

The DNA of lymphomas from the 21 AKXD tumor strains was analyzed for the presence of somatically acquired ecotropic and MCF proviruses (Mucenski ***et al.***, 1987b; Gilbert ***et al.***, unpublished results). Among the lymphomas analyzed, the majority (approximately 80%) contained somatically acquired proviruses. Lymphomas not containing somatic proviruses may represent polyclonal tumors, rare spontaneous nonvirally induced tumors, or tumors containing proviral sequences not detectable with the hybridization probes used. Most tumors appeared to be monoclonal in origin. These findings are consistent with the hypothesis that these tumors are induced by retroviruses.

Table 3. Distribution of lymphoma types within 21 AKXD RI strains

AKXD RI Strain	Predominant Lymphoma Type
6,17,21,24,26	T cell
2,11,13,14,27	B cell
23	Myeloid
3,7,8,9,10,12, 15,16,18,22	T and B cell

Table 4. Cellular genes activated by viral integration in AKXD lymphomas

Lymphoma Type	Number of Lymphomas	Locus						
		Myc	*Pvt-1*	*Fis-1*	*Pim-1*	***Myb***	***Mlvi-1***	***Mlvi-2***
T cell	111	21	5	4	14	0	5	2
B cell	119	0	0	0	4	0	0	0
Myeloid	9	0	0	0	0	0	0	0

MCF proviruses were detected primarily in T-cell lymphomas, whereas ecotropic proviruses were detected in lymphomas of B cell and myeloid lineages. These results suggest a model to account for the variation in lymphoma types observed in different AKXD strains. The model suggests that, during inbreeding, the AKXD strains segregated for several genes, including proviruses, that affect the nature of recombinant viruses formed in preleukemic animals. The different recombinant viruses have different oncogenic potential.

Known Cellular Genes Activated by Viral Integration in AKXD Lymphomas

The large number of well-characterized AKXD lymphomas representing many diverse pathological types provides a valuable database for identifying cellular loci activated by viral integration in tumors and for determining whether the repertoire of cellular genes activated by viral integration in tumors varies with respect to cell type. In an initial series of studies, 239 AKXD lymphomas of T cell, B cell, or myeloid origin were screened for virally induced rearrangements in seven loci previously shown to be activated by viral integration in other murine or rat lymphomas (Mucenski *et al.*, 1987a) (Table 4). Virally induced rearrangements were detected in six of the loci, ***Myc***, ***Pvt-1***, ***Pim-1***, ***Mlvi-1***, ***Mlvi-2***, and ***Fis-1***. No rearrangements were detected in the ***Myb*** locus. This was not surprising since viral integrations in the ***Myb*** locus in murine hematopoietic tumors have been observed only in myeloid tumors and only 9 of the 239 AKXD lymphomas analyzed were of myeloid origin.

Nearly 90% of the rearrangements were detected in T-cell lymphomas. Only a few rearrangements were detected in B-cell lymphomas and these rearrangements occurred specifically in the ***Pim-1*** locus. No rearrangements were detected in myeloid tumors.

Seven lymphomas contained rearrangements in two different loci, suggesting that rearrangements in different protooncogene loci within the same tumor cell population can act in concert to achieve neoplastic transformation. Tumors possessing multiple rearrangements may thus provide important information about genes that can act cooperatively to induce neoplastic disease. Overall, these results suggest that the repertoire of cellular protooncogenes activated by viral integration in tumors is different for each hematopoietic cell type.

Evi-1: A New Common Viral Integration Site Identified in DNA of AKXD-23 Myeloid Tumors

AKXD-23 mice develop myeloid tumors at high frequency (70% incidence) unlike other AKXD strains that develop B-cell lymphomas, T-cell lymphomas, or both. The myeloid tumors that develop in AKXD-23 mice appear very late in life (415 ± 19 days). AKXD-23 myeloid tumors are monoclonal and their DNA contains somatically acquired ecotropic proviruses, suggesting that they are retrovirally induced.

Among the AKXD-23 tumor DNAs examined for somatically acquired proviruses, most, if not all, appeared to contain a provirus integrated into the same chromosomal domain. Representative Southern blot results for tumor DNAs isolated from spleen, cleaved with ***Eco*RI**, and hybridized with an ecotropic virus-specific envelope probe, are shown in Fig. 1. Brain DNA, which is usually not infiltrated with large amounts of tumor tissue, was included as a control to discriminate between endogenous and somatically acquired ecotropic proviruses. Ecotropic proviruses are not cleaved by ***Eco*RI**, so the size of the fragments detected on Southern blots depends upon where ***Eco*RI** cleavage sites are located in flanking cellular DNA. AKXD-23 mice carry two endogenous ecotropic proviral loci, ***Emv-11*** and ***Emv-14***. These proviruses generate ***Eco*RI** fragments of 11.4- and 25.0-kilobases (kb) in size (Fig. 1). In addition, a 16.4-kb fragment was detected in each tumor DNA (Fig. 1). The 16.4-kb fragment was either not detected or only faintly detected in brain DNA; this faint hybridization is thought to reflect the infiltration of small numbers of tumor cells into brain tissue. These results strongly suggest that each tumor contains a somatically acquired ecotropic provirus integrated into the same chromosomal domain. This potential common viral integration site was designated ***Evi-1*** (ecotropic viral integration site-1).

To confirm the existence of a common viral integration site, one of the 16.4-kb ***Eco*RI** proviral DNA-cellular DNA junction fragments was molecularly cloned and unique sequence flanking cellular DNA probes were isolated (Mucenski ***et al.***, 1988b). ***Eco*RI** digested DNAs from AKXD lymphomas were then screened for rearrangements in the ***Evi-1*** locus (Table 5). Virally induced rearrangements were detected in the ***Evi-1*** locus in all nine AKXD myeloid tumors analyzed including the seven myeloid tumors obtained from AKXD-23 mice. ***Evi-1*** rearrangements were not detected in T-cell lymphomas. A few ***Evi-1*** rearrangements were detected in B-cell tumors. These results confirm that ***Evi-1*** is a common integration site in AKXD tumors. The distribution of ***Evi-1*** rearrangements among the three classes of

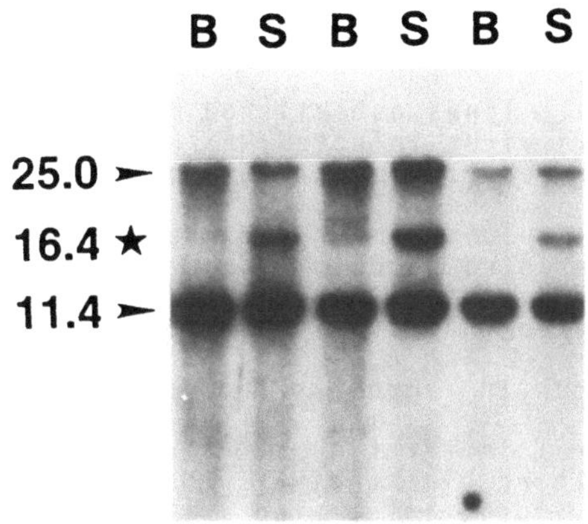

Fig. 1. Common Site of Viral Integration in AKXD-23 Myeloid Tumors

Ten μg of DNA from brain (B) and lymphomatous spleen (S) of three AKXD-23 animals was digested to completion with *Eco*RI, submitted to Southern blot analysis, and hybridized with an ecotropic virus-specific envelope probe as described (Mucenski *et al.*, 1988a). Fragment sizes were calculated using ^{32}P-labelled *Hind*III-digested lambda DNA fragments loaded in a parallel lane of the same gel.

Table 5. Correlation between *Evi-1* rearrangements and lymphoma type

Tumor Origin	Lymphoma Type[a]		
	B cell	T cell	Myeloid
AKXD	2/67	0/54	9/9
NFS/N	0/4	0/4	7/44

[a]Number positive/number typed.

lymphomas was different than the distribution previously observed with *Myc*, *Pvt-1*, *Fis-1*, *Pim-1*, *Mlvi-1*, and *Mlvi-2* (Table 4). This result further supports the hypothesis that the repertoire of cellular genes activated by viral integration in tumors varies according to tumor cell type.

Evi-1 Rearrangements are Detected in Myeloid Tumors and Cell Lines From Strains Other Than AKXD

DNA from tumors and cell lines established from hematopoietic neoplasms that arose in virus-infected NFS/N or NFS/N-hybrid mice were also screened for rearrangements in the *Evi-1* locus (Mucenski ***et al.***, 1988b) (Table 5). Rearrangements were detected in 7 of 44 (16%) DNAs from these myeloid tumors and myeloid cell lines. No rearrangements were detected in DNAs from T-cell or B-cell lines. These findings are consistent with previous results obtained with AKXD lymphomas indicating that *Evi-1* rearrangements occur primarily in myeloid tumors. These findings also indicate that rearrangements in the Evi-1 locus occur in lymphomas from strains other than AKXD.

The location of proviral integration sites within the *Evi-1* locus was determined by Southern blot analysis (Mucenski ***et al.***, 1988b). The nature of the proviruses integrated into the *Evi-1* locus (ecotropic or MCF) was also determined. All rearrangements within the *Evi-1* locus in the AKXD lymphomas were due to the integration of ecotropic viruses. All viral integrations occurred within a 0.6-kb region. Most viral integrations were clustered within a 300-base-pair region. All proviruses had the same transcriptional orientation. Similar results were found for cell lines and myeloid tumors obtained from NFS/N or NFS/N-hybrid mice.

Evi-1 Maps to Mouse Chromosome 3 and Represents a Newly Identified Locus in the Mouse

One method to determine if *Evi-1* is homologous to any previously identified protooncogene, growth factor, growth factor receptor, or common integration site is to hybridize molecular clones representative of these loci to *Evi-1* sequences. However, this approach has certain limitations. First, the exact 5′ and 3′ boundaries of these genes are not all known and, consequently, *Evi-1*-hybridizing sequences may not be represented in these clones. Second, these loci may be large and the probe representing *Evi-1* may be in a large intron. Third, viral integration may affect transcription of flanking genes over large distances. An alternative and more powerful approach is to map the chromosomal location of the *Evi-1* locus in the mouse to determine if it is distinct from other already mapped loci. The chromosomal location of *Evi-1* was determined by standard genetic techniques (Mucenski ***et al.***, 1988a). These studies showed that *Evi-1* maps to mouse chromosome 3 and is distinct from all other loci previously mapped on chromosome 3. These findings suggest that *Evi-1* represents a novel locus involved in myeloid disease.

Evi-1 Encodes a Zinc Finger Protein That is Evolutionarily Well Conserved

Sequences from the *Evi-1* locus are well evolutionarily conserved (Buchberg ***et al.***, unpublished results). This result is expected for a gene that has an important function in development, normal cell processes, or both. Transcripts from the *Evi-1* locus have recently been identified (Morishita, Parker, Mucenski, Jenkins, Copeland and Ihle, manuscript submitted). Viral integrations in the *Evi-1* locus activate transcription of this gene; transcripts were not detected in normal myeloid cells. DNA sequencing studies indicated that this gene is a member of the ***Kruppel*** family of zinc finger proteins. A number of these proteins have been shown to be DNA binding proteins that are capable of regulating gene expression in ***trans***. This represents the first demonstration of the retroviral activation of a gene encoding a zinc finger protein and the first implication for a member of this gene family in the transformation of hematopoietic cells.

Evi-1 is Closely Linked to the *Fim-3* Common Integration Site

A common integration site, ***Fim-3***, was identified in F-MuLV-induced myeloblastic leukemias (Bordereaux ***et al.***, 1987). Interspecific chromosome mapping studies indicated that ***Evi-1*** is tightly linked to ***Fim-3*** (Bartholomew, Morishita, Buchberg, Jenkins, Copeland, and Ihle, manuscript in preparation). No recombinants were observed in 151 interspecific backcross animals analyzed. Restriction mapping and hybridization studies of approximately 50-kb of the ***Fim-3*** locus failed to demonstrate overlapping regions with the ***Evi-1*** locus. However, viral integrations in the ***Fim-3*** locus in NFS/N myeloid tumor cell lines activated transcription of the ***Evi-1*** locus in the absence of viral integrations in ***Evi-1***. Viral transcripts from the ***Fim-3*** locus have not been identified. These findings suggest that ***Evi-1*** and ***Fim-3*** represent two independent common viral integration sites that activate transcription of the same gene.

BXH-2 RECOMBINANT INBRED MICE: POTENTIAL MODEL FOR HUMAN ACUTE MYELOID LEUKEMIA

BXH-2 RI mice spontaneously express an ecotropic MuLV beginning early in life and die of granulocytic leukemia (with nearly a 100 percent incidence) by one year of age (average age of onset is 7 months) (Bedigian ***et al.***, 1981; 1984; Jenkins ***et al.***, 1982a). The virus is not encoded in the BXH-2 germline but is transmitted horizontally in this strain. The high virus expression and high tumor incidence in BXH-2 mice are traits not characteristic of the BXH-2 progenitor strains (C57BL/6J and C3H/HeJ) or of the 11 other BXH RI strains.

High virus expression in BXH-2 mice appears causally associated with the high tumor incidence in this strain. When the BXH-2 ecotropic virus was injected into newborn mice of several other BXH RI strains, myeloid leukemia developed at high frequency (Bedigian ***et al.***, 1984). Southern blot analysis of BXH-2 tumor DNAs indicated that the tumors are monoclonal and contain somatically acquired ecotropic proviruses (Bedigian ***et al.***, 1984; Buchberg, Mucenski, Bedigian, Jenkins, and Copeland, manuscript in preparation). Somatically acquired MCF proviruses were seldom observed in tumor DNA. These findings suggest that BXH-2 myeloid disease is induced by integration of ecotropic viruses.

Ecotropic Viral Integration in BXH-2 Tumors Does Not Appear to Activate the Expression of Known Cellular Genes

Several known cellular genes that may be involved in BXH-2 tumorigenesis were characterized by Southern blot analysis to determine if they were rearranged in BXH-2 myeloid tumors (Buchberg ***et al.***, manuscript in preparation) (Table 6). In general, virally induced rearrangements were not detected. However, three rearrangements were detected in the ***Myb*** locus in 65 BXH-2 tumors analyzed. Further restriction analysis indicated that these rearrangements were not due to ecotropic viral integration. The

Table 6. Absence of virally-induced rearrangements in a number of cellular genes in BXH-2 myeloid tumors

Gene Family	Locus
Protooncogene	***Myc*, *Myb***, p53
Growth Factor	***Il-3*, *Csfgm*, *Csfg*, *Csfm***
Growth Factor Receptor	***Fms***
Common Integration Site	***Fim-1*, *Fim-2*, *Fim-3*, *Evi-1*, *Fis-1*, *Pim-1*, *Pvt-1***

nature of these rearrangements remains to be determined. Surprisingly, ***Evi-1*** rearrangements were not detected in BXH-2 tumors even though they were identified in 100 percent of AKXD myeloid tumors analyzed. This suggests that the repertoire of cellular genes activated by viral integration in myeloid tumors of BXH-2 and AKXD mice differs.

Evi-2: A New Common Integration Site Identified in BXH-2 Myeloid Tumors

In order to identify the genes that are activated by viral integration in BXH-2 myeloid tumors, somatically acquired ecotropic proviruses along with flanking host sequences were molecularly cloned from BXH-2 tumors and analyzed to determine if they represented common viral integration sites. A common viral integration site, designated ***Evi-2***, was identified in BXH-2 myeloid tumors (Buchberg ***et al.***, manuscript in preparation). Rearrangements in the ***Evi-2*** locus were detected in 11 of 65 (17%) BXH-2 myeloid tumors analyzed. Chromosome mapping studies indicated that ***Evi-2*** is located on mouse chromosome 11 and is distinct from all other loci mapped on mouse chromosome 11 (Buchberg ***et al.***, 1988). This finding suggests that ***Evi-2*** is a novel locus involved in BXH-2 myeloid tumorigenesis.

Two ***Evi-2*** transcripts of 1.6- and 2.4-kb in size have been identified in several normal adult mouse tissues (Buchberg ***et al.***, unpublished results). ***Evi-2*** sequences are evolutionarily well conserved and have been identified in human DNA. Preliminary mapping studies indicate that human ***Evi-2***-related sequences map to human chromosome 17, band q11-q12 (M. LeBeau, personal communication). Future studies will be required to determine if ***Evi-2*** is causally associated with any of the genetic disorders mapping to human chromosome 17. One very interesting candidate gene is the gene that is associated with the chromosome 17 breakpoint in the 15:17 translocation chromosome. The breakpoint of this translocation on chromosome 17 is in band q12-q21, the same region where ***Evi-2*** has been mapped. This translocation is identified in nearly 100 per cent of human acute promyelocytic leukemias (Rowley ***et al.***, 1977a,b).

FUTURE PROSPECTS

The studies presented here demonstrate the value of recombinant inbred strains for studying the molecular genetic basis of murine hematopoietic tumors and for identifying novel loci involved in mouse and, potentially, human disease. The somatically acquired proviruses identified in these tumors should prove valuable for identifying new genes involved not only in myeloid disease but in T-cell and B-cell disease as well.

ACKNOWLEDGEMENTS

We thank Linda Brubaker for typing this manuscript. This research was supported by the National Cancer Institute under Contract No. NO1-CO-74101 with Bionetics Research, Inc.

REFERENCES

Baumbach WR, Stanley ER, Cole MD (1987) Induction of clonal monocyte-macrophage tumors ***in vivo*** by a mouse c-***myc*** retrovirus: Rearrangement of the CSF-1 gene as a secondary transforming event. Mol Cell Biol 7: 664-671

Bedigian HG, Johnson DA, Jenkins NA, Copeland NG, Evans R (1984) Spontaneous and induced leukemias of myeloid origin in recombinant inbred BXH mice. J Virol 51: 586-594

Bedigian HG, Taylor BA, Meier H (1981) Expression of murine leukemia viruses in the highly lymphomatous BXH-2 recombinant inbred mouse strain. J Virol 39: 632-640

Bordereaux D, Fichelson S, Sola B, Tambourin PE, Gisselbrecht S (1987) Frequent involvement of the ***fim-3*** region in Friend murine leukemia virus-induced mouse myeloblastic leukemias. J Virol 61: 4043-4045

Buchberg AM, Bedigian HG, Taylor BA, Brownell E, Ihle JN, Nagata S, Jenkins NA, Copeland NG (1988) Localization of ***Evi-2*** to chromosome 11: Linkage to other proto-oncogene and growth factor loci using interspecific backcross mice. Oncogene Res 2: 149-165

Copeland NG, Jenkins NA, Nexo B, Schultz AM, Rein A, Mikkelsen T, Jorgensen P (1988) Poorly expressed endogenous ecotropic provirus of DBA/2 mice encodes a mutant $Pr65^{gag}$ protein that is not myristylated. J Virol 62: 479-487

Corcoran LM, Adams JM, Dunn AR, Cory S (1984) Murine T lymphomas in which the cellular ***myc*** oncogene has been activated by retroviral insertion. Cell 37: 113-122

Cuypers HT, Selten G, Quint W, Zijlstra M, Maandag ER, Boelens W, van Wezenbeek P, Melief C, Berns A (1984) Murine leukemia virus-induced T-cell lymphomagenesis: Integration of proviruses in a distinct chromosomal region. Cell 37: 141-150

George DL, Glick B, Trusko S, Freeman N (1986) Enhanced c-Ki-***ras*** expression associated with Friend virus integration in a bone marrow-derived mouse cell line. Proc Natl Acad Sci USA 83: 1651-1655

Gisselbrecht S, Fichelson S, Sola B, Bordereaux D, Hampe A, Andre C, Galibert F, Tambourin P (1987) Frequent c-***fms*** activation by proviral insertion in mouse myeloblastic leukemias. Nature 329: 259-261

Graham M, Adams JM, Cory S (1985) Murine T lymphomas with retroviral inserts in the chromosomal 15 locus for plasmacytoma variant translocations. Nature 314: 740-743

Gross L (1983) In: Oncogenic Viruses, Vol 1 (3rd edition) Pergamon Press, Inc., Elmsford, New York

Hanecak R, Pattengale PK, Fan H (1988) Addition or substitution of simian virus 40 enhancer sequences into the Moloney murine leukemia virus (M-MuLV) long terminal repeat yields infectious M-MuLV with altered biological properties. J Virol 62: 2427-2436

Hartley JW, Wolford NK, Old LJ, Rowe WP (1977) A new class of murine leukemia virus associated with development of spontaneous lymphomas. Proc Natl Acad Sci USA 74: 789-792

Herr W, Gilbert W (1983) Somatically acquired recombinant murine leukemia proviruses in thymic leukemias of AKR/J mice. J Virol 46: 70-82

Herr W, Gilbert W (1984) Free and integrated recombinant murine leukemia virus DNAs appear in preleukemic thymuses of AKR/J mice. J Virol 50: 155-162

Holland CA, Hartley JW, Rowe WP, Hopkins N (1985) At least four viral genes contribute to the leukemogenicity of murine retrovirus MCF 247 in AKR mice. J Virol 53: 158-165

Jenkins NA, Copeland NG, Taylor BA, Bedigian HG, Lee BK (1982a) Ecotropic murine leukemia virus DNA content of normal and lymphomatous tissues of BXH-2 recombinant inbred mice. J Virol 42: 379-388

Jenkins NA, Copeland NG, Taylor BA, Lee BK (1982b) Organization, distribution, and stability of endogenous ecotropic murine leukemia virus DNA sequences in chromosomes of ***Mus musculus***. J Virol 43: 26-36

Li Y, Holland CA, Hartley JW, Hopkins N (1984) Viral integrations near c-***myc*** in 10-20% of MCF 247-induced AKR lymphomas. Proc Natl Acad Sci USA 81: 6808-6811

Marth JD, Peet R, Krebs EG, Perlmutter RM (1985) A lymphocyte-specific protein-tyrosine kinase gene is rearranged and overexpressed in the murine T cell lymphoma LSTRA. Cell 43: 393-404

Moreau-Gachelin F, Tavitian A, Tambourin P (1988) ***Spi-1*** is a putative oncogene in virally induced murine erythroleukaemias. Nature 331: 277-280

Mucenski ML, Gilbert DJ, Taylor BA, Jenkins NA, Copeland NG (1987a) Common sites of viral integration in lymphomas arising in AKXD recombinant inbred mouse strains. Oncogene Res 2: 33-48

Mucenski ML, Taylor BA, Copeland NG, Jenkins NA (1987b) Characterization of somatically acquired ecotropic and mink cell focus-forming viruses in lymphomas of AKXD recombinant inbred mice. J Virol 61: 2929-2933

Mucenski ML, Taylor BA, Copeland NG, Jenkins NA (1988a) Chromosomal location of ***Evi-1***, a common site of ecotropic viral integration in AKXD murine myeloid tumors. Oncogene Res 2: 219-233

Mucenski ML, Taylor BA, Ihle JN, Hartley JW, Morse HC III, Jenkins NA, Copeland NG (1988b) Identification of a common ecotropic viral integration site, ***Evi-1***, in the DNA of AKXD murine myeloid tumors. Mol Cell Biol 8: 301-308

Mucenski ML, Taylor BA, Jenkins NA, Copeland NG (1986) AKXD recombinant inbred strains: models for studying the molecular genetic basis of murine lymphomas. Mol Cell Biol 6: 4236-4243

Mushinski JF, Potter M, Bauer SR, Reddy EP (1983) DNA rearrangement and altered RNA expression of the c-***myb*** oncogene in mouse plasmacytoid lymphosarcomas. Science 220: 795-798

Nusse R (1986) The activation of cellular oncogenes by retroviral insertion. Trends in Genet 2: 244-247

Quint W, Boelens W, van Wezenbeek P, Cuypers T, Maandag ER, Selten G, Berns A (1984) Generation of AKR mink cell focus-forming viruses: A conserved single copy xenotropic-like provirus provides recombinant long terminal repeat sequences. J Virol 50: 432-438

Reicin A, Yang J-Q, Marcu KB, Fleissner E, Koehne CF, O'Donnell PV (1986) Deregulation of the c-***myc*** oncogene in virus-induced thymic lymphomas of AKR/J mice. Mol Cell Biol 6: 4088-4092

Rowley JD, Golomb HM, Dougherty C (1977a) 15/17 translocation, a consistent chromosomal change in acute promyelocytic leukemia. Lancet 1: 549-550

Rowley JD, Golomb HM, Vardman J, Fukuhara S, Dougherty C, Potter D. (1977b) Further evidence for a non-random chromosomal abnormality in acute promyelocytic leukemia. Int J Cancer 20: 869-872

Selten G, Cuypers HT, Berns A (1985) Proviral activation of the putative oncogene ***Pim-1*** in MuLV-induced T-cell lymphomas. EMBO J 4: 1793-1798

Selten G, Cuypers HT, Boelens W, Robanus-Maandag E, Verbeek J, Domen J, van Beveren C, Berns A (1986) The primary structure of the putative oncogene ***Pim-1*** shows extensive homology with protein kinases. Cell 46: 603-611

Selten G, Cuypers HT, Zijlstra M, Melief C, Berns A (1984) Involvement of c-***myc*** in MuLV-induced T cell lymphomas in mice: Frequency and mechanisms of activation. EMBO J 3: 3215-3222

Shen-Ong GLC, Morse HC III, Potter M, Mushinski JF (1986) Two modes of c-***myb*** activation in virus-induced mouse myeloid tumors. Mol Cell Biol 6: 380-392.

Shen-Ong GLC, Potter M, Mushinski JF, Lavu S, Reddy EP (1984) Activation of the c-***myb*** locus by viral insertional mutagenesis in plasmacytoid lymphosarcomas. Science 226: 1077-1080

Silver J, Kozak C (1986) Common proviral integration region on mouse chromosome 7 in lymphomas and myelogenous leukemias induced by Friend murine leukemia virus. J Virol 57: 526-533.

Sola B, Fichelson S, Bordereaux D, Tambourin PE, Gisselbrecht S (1986) ***fim-1*** and ***fim-2***: Two new integration regions of Friend murine leukemia virus in myeloblastic leukemias. J Virol 60: 718-725

Taylor BA (1979) Recombinant inbred strains: Use in gene mapping. In: Morse HC III (ed) Origins of inbred mice. Academic Press, Inc., New York

Villemur R, Monczak Y, Rassart E, Kozak C, Jolicoeur P (1987) Identification of a new common provirus integration site in Gross passage A murine leukemia virus-induced mouse thymoma DNA. Mol Cell Biol 7: 512-522

Voronova AF, Sefton BM (1986) Expression of a new tyrosine protein kinase is stimulated by retrovirus promoter insertion. Nature 319: 682-685

Warren W, Lawley PD, Gardner E, Harris G, Ball JK, Cooper CS (1987) Induction of thymomas by N-methyl-N-nitrosourea in AKR mice: Interaction between the chemical carcinogen and endogenous murine leukemia viruses. Carcinogenesis 8: 163-172

Weinstein Y, Ihle JN, Lavu S, Reddy EP (1986) Truncation of the c-***myb*** gene by a retroviral integration in an interleukin 3-dependent myeloid leukemia cell line. Proc Natl Acad Sci USA 83:5010-5014

Wirschubsky Z, Tschilis P, Klein G, Sumegi J (1986) Rearrangement of c-***myc***, ***Pim-1*** and ***Mlvi-1*** and trisomy of chromosome 15 in MCF- and Moloney-MuLV-induced murine T-cell leukemias. Int J Cancer 38: 739-745

Mechanisms in the Transformation of IL3-Dependent Hematopoietic Stem Cells

J.N. Ihle[1,2], K. Morishita[1], D.S. Parker, C. Bartholomew[1], D. Askew[1], A. Buchberg, N.A. Jenkins, N. Copeland and Y. Weinstein[3]

BRI-Basic Research Program, NCI-Frederick Cancer Research Facility, Frederick, Maryland 21701

INTRODUCTION

The hematopoietic system is derived from the progeny of pluripotential stem cells which can differentiate along lymphoid or myeloid lineages (Keller et al.1985; Williams et al.1984; Joyner et al.1983; Lemischka et al.1986). Interleukin 3 (IL3) is a T cell derived lymphokine which supports the proliferation and differentiation of early hematopoietic stem cells _in vitro_ and has been speculated to play a comparable role _in vivo_ (Ihle, and Weinstein, 1986; Ihle, 1988). A role for IL3 in the mechanisms by which retroviruses induce leukemias has been hypothesized based on several observations. Initially it was observed that there was a correlation between a T cell immune response to retroviruses and the latency and frequency of leukemias (Lee et al.1981a). It was subsequently demonstrated that the T cell response consisted, in part, of viral antigen specific helper T cells which produced IL3 following antigenic stimulation (Lee, and Ihle, 1981b). As a consequence of this immune response there is a dramatic increase in the cells proliferating in response to IL3 _in vivo_ (Lee, and Ihle, 1981) which has been hypothesized to constitute an increased pool of progenitors for transformation.

A role for IL3 in leukemogenesis has been further suggested by the observation that the majority of retrovirus induced myeloid leukemias are dependent on IL3 for growth. In particular, Moloney MuLV (MoLV) (Ihle et al.1984) or Lake Cascitus wild mouse ecotropic virus (CasBrM MuLV) (Holmes et al.1985) induced myeloid leukemias require IL3 for growth _in vitro_. Using IL3 as a growth factor it has been possible to isolate a number of myeloid leukemia cell lines. These cells retain an absolute requirement for IL3 and rapidly lose viability in the absence of IL3. The cells have varying abilities to respond to other hematopoietic growth factors and express myeloid lineage markers of various stages of differentiation. Because of their absolute requirement for growth factors, these myeloid leukemia cell lines have been useful for studies of IL3 signal transduction.

The transformation of hematopoietic cells can involve an alteration in the growth factor requirements of the cells, an altered ability to terminally differentiate or both. The properties of IL3-dependent myeloid leukemia cell lines indicate that transformation has primarily affected the ability of the cells to terminally differentiate. Although expressing phenotypic properties associated with early myel-

---

1.) Current address: Department of Biochemistry, St. Jude Children's Hospital, 332 North Lauderdale, Memphis, Tennessee, 38101

2.) To whom requests should be addressed.

3.) Department of Microbiology and Immunology, Ben Gurion University of the Negev, Beer Sheva, Israel

Current Topics in Microbiology and Immunology, Vol. 149

oid differentiation, the cells do not spontaneously differentiate nor do the cells differentiate in response to various chemical inducers or hematopoietic growth factors. The identification of the genes associated with this type of transformation may provide insights into the genes involved in the regulation of normal differentiation.

Transformation by retroviruses is often due to the integration of the viruses into or near cellular genes whose altered expression can affect the properties of the cells. To determine the types of genes associated with the transformation of IL3-dependent myeloid cells, we have examined IL3-dependent myeloid leukemia cell lines for viral integrations in known oncogenes or common sites of viral integrations. Among a variety of the transforming genes, only the myb gene was found to be activated in IL3-dependent cell lines (Weinstein et al.1986; Weinstein et al.1987). Among the common sites of retroviral integration, the Evi-1 locus was found to contain proviruses in a number of the cell lines (Mucenski et al.1988). Characterization of expression from the Evi-1 locus has demonstrated that viral integrations are associated with the activation of the expression of a gene encoding a Zinc finger protein.

EXPERIMENTAL RESULTS

Isolation and Characteristics of IL3-Dependent Myeloid Leukemia Cells

A variety of IL3-dependent cell lines have been established from MoLV (DA series) or CasBrM MuLV (NFS series) induced myeloid leukemias. The designation and properties of a few of these cell lines are shown in table 1. All the lines require IL3 for maintenance of viability and/or proliferation. In addition the lines show variable responses to other hematopoietic growth factors. Although not indicated, the responses to other growth factors are generally less than or equal to those seen with IL3. In addition the cell lines express phenotypic markers of early myeloid lineage differentiation although to varying extents. In general it has not been possible to establish a clear correlation between the growth factor responses and specific patterns of expression of lineage markers. All the lines have morphologies of early myeloid lineage cells and show little or no spontaneous differentiation.

Table 1. Phenotypic Properties of IL3-Dependent Cell Lines

Cell Line	Growth Factor Responses					Phenotypic Markers			
Designation	IL3	IL4	IL6	G-CSF	GM-CSF	Thy-1	8C5	MPO	Mac-1
DA-1	+[a]	-	-	-	+	4%[b]	<1%	ND	77%
DA-3	+	+	-	-	+	95%	25%	+	40%
DA-13	+	+	-	-	+	95%	<1%	ND	<1%
DA-34	+	+	-	-	+	95%	<1%	ND	<1%
NFS-58	+	-	-	-	-	90%	37%	+	50%
NFS-60	+	-	+	+	-	90%	20%	+	<4%
NFS-78	+	-	-	-	-	83%	10%	ND	40%
NFS-107	+	+	-	-	-	<1%	23%	+	62%

a Responses to the indicated hematopoietic growth factors were determined by ^{3}H thymidine incorporation assays.

b Expression of various cell surface markers was determined by FACS analysis (Thy-1, 8C5, Mac-1) or by Northern analysis (MPO).

Myb Gene Rearrangements in the IL3-Dependent NFS-60 Myeloid Line.

To determine the genes involved in the transformation of IL3-dependent myeloid cells, we examined the lines for viral insertions in known oncogenes. No rearrangements were detected in the K-ras, N-ras, H-ras, mos, abl, ets-1, ets-2, N-myc, L-myc, or c-raf proto-oncogenes. However, one cell line (NFS-60) contained a rearrangement of the c-myb gene. This was of particular interest because the v-myb gene has been shown to cause the transformation of myeloid lineage cells and to specifically alter the ability of the cells to differentiate without altering their growth factor requirements (Beug et al.1982; Moscovici et al.1983). For this reason the c-myb rearrangement was further characterized.

As illustrated in figure 1 and previously described in detail (Weinstein et al.1986), the rearrangement involved the integration of a complete CasBrM MuLV retrovirus into a 1.5 kb EcoRI fragment. This genomic fragment contains the sixth viral related c-myb exon which encodes sequences found in the middle of c-myb. From the structure of the integration, transcription from the rearranged locus should result in a truncated transcript of approximately 2 kb which terminates in the 5' viral LTR at the transcriptional termination site of the virus. As previously illustrated, the major transcript detected in NFS-60 cells is a 2 kb transcript while the normal 4 kb transcript is present at much lower levels. Since NFS-60 cells retain one normal allele and cells at a comparable stage of differentiation normally express c-myb, the predominance of the truncated transcript indicates that the integrated provirus also effects the levels of transcription of the locus or stability of the RNA.

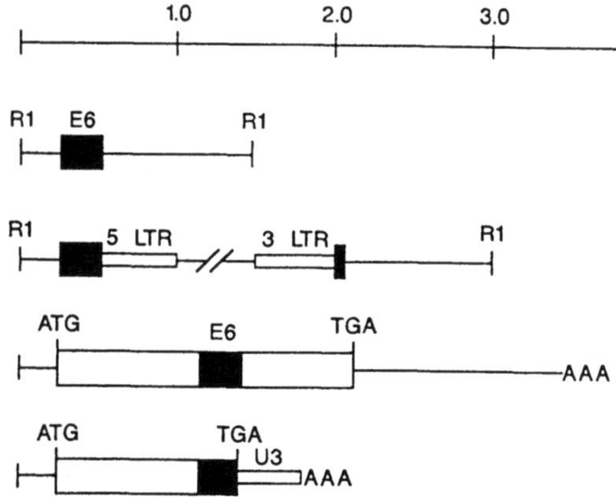

Fig. 1. Structure of Viral Integration Site in the c-myb gene in NFS-60 cells. The structure of the integration site was deduced by sequencing of genomic clones and the structure of the RNAs were deduced by sequencing of cDNA clones. Exon E6 corresponds to the sixth cellular exon defined by the sequence of the avian v-myb transforming gene. The U3 sequences are derived from the 5' LTR of the integrated provirus.

We also examined NFS-60 cells for c-myb protein using an antiserum against the amino region of the myb gene. From the structure of the integrated provirus and from sequencing of cDNA clones, it would be predicted that translation would terminate at the juncture of the c-*myb* and LTR sequences at a translational terminator which is introduced by the first three bases of the viral LTR in-frame to the coding sequence of the c-*myb* gene. Consistent with this prediction, the major protein detected by immunoprecipitation is a 45 kd nuclear protein (data not shown). As predicted from the Northern analysis the normal 90 kd c-*myb* protein was present at much lower levels than the truncated gene product.

Taken together the results demonstrate that in NFS-60 cells, a retroviral insertion into the c-*myb* locus resulted in the overproduction of a truncated transcript and a carboxyl-truncated protein. Strikingly, the carboxyl truncation occurred in the region of the carboxyl truncations which were associated with the transduction of the avian c-*myb* gene into the myeloid lineage transforming viruses AMV and E26 (Klempnauer et al.1982; Klempnauer et al.1983). Unlike the transforming viruses however, we have not detected any rearrangements in the 5' or amino terminal region of the gene comparable to the amino terminal deletions which are present in the avian transforming viruses. These results suggest that the carboxyl-truncations are sufficient for the acquisition of transforming potential.

Insertions in the Evi-1 Common Site of Integration.

Because of the paucity of rearrangements of known oncogenes in IL3-dependent myeloid leukemia cell lines we have also examined the lines for viral integrations in a number of common integration sites. In particular the lines were examined for integrations in *Fim*-1, *Fim*-2, *Evi*-1, *Evi*-2, *Mlvi*-1, *Mlvi*-2, *Pim*-1 and *Pim*-2. Among these, viral integrations in the *Evi*-1 locus were found in three IL3-dependent cell lines (NFS-60, NFS-48, NFS-78) (Mucenski et al.1988). Because of the frequency of viral integrations in this locus we further characterized the locus and identified its associated gene.

Initially, additional genomic clones were isolated and a more detailed restriction map of the locus was developed which spanned approximately 28 kb of the locus. Examination of IL3-dependent cell lines for rearrangements outside of the 7 kb EcoRI fragment which defined the *Evi*-1 locus demonstrated that two additional lines (DA-1, NFS-58) contained retroviral integrations in a 5 kb EcoRI fragment flanking the 7 kb fragment.

The Evi-1 Locus Encodes a Member of the Zinc Finger Family.

To determine whether viral integrations had altered transcription of a gene associated with the *Evi*-1 locus, various genomic probes were used in Northern hybridizations. Using a probe which spanned the integration sites in NFS-60, NFS-78 and NFS-48, a low level of transcripts were detected in NFS-78 cells. This probe was used to isolated cDNA clones from a lambda gt10 library made from polyA+ RNA from NFS-78 cells. The structures of two cDNA clones were determined by restriction mapping and sequencing and consisted of viral and cellular sequences as shown in figure 2 and previously described in detail (Morishita et al.1988). The transcript from which one clone was isolated initiated in the virus and transcription continued through the 3' LTR into cellular sequences. In the second case the RNA had spliced out of the virus and into cellular sequences. The sequence of the cellular cDNA sequences relative to the sequence derived from genomic clones indicated the presence of two potential cellular exons.

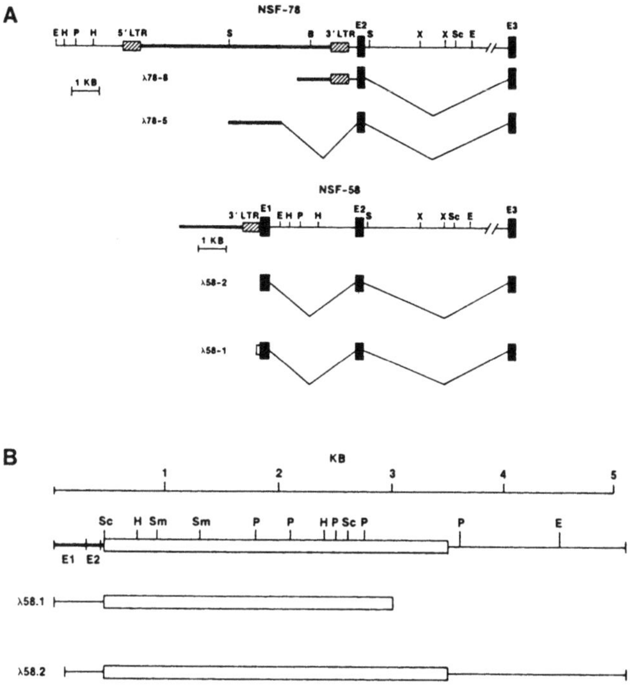

Fig. 2. Structure of Evi-1 cDNA Clones from NFS-78 and NFS-58 Cells. The structures of the cDNA clones were deduced by partial sequencing or complete sequencing of cDNA clones.

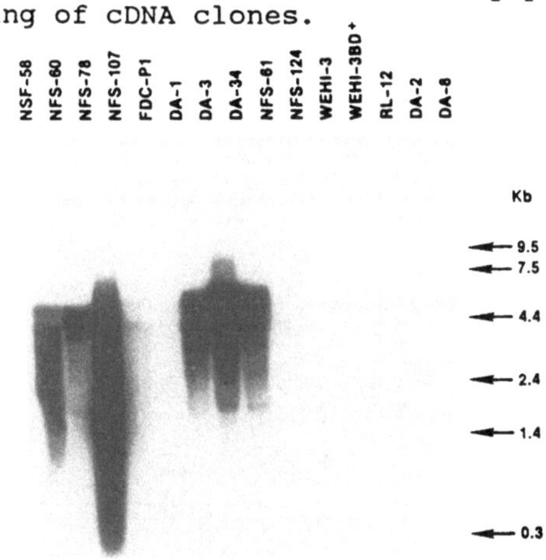

Fig. 3. Expression of Evi-1 Transcripts in Cell Lines Containing Viral Integrations in the Evi-1 Locus or the CB-1/Fim-3 Locus. PolyA+ RNAs were prepared from the indicated lines by standard procedures and were resolved by electrophoresis on 0.8% agarose cells following denaturation with glyoxal. The RNAs were transferred to nitrocellulose and the filters hybridized with the NFS 58.2 cDNA clone.

Because of the complexity of the cDNAs, probes for the cellular exon sequences were used to isolate additional cDNA clones from a lambda gt10 library made with polyA+ RNA from NFS-58 cells. The structure of these clones is shown in figure 2. In one clone there were 12 bp derived from a viral 3' LTR while the second clone contained no viral sequences. Because of the lack of viral sequences the second clone was used to further characterize transcripts from the locus. As shown in figure 3, cell lines containing rearrangements in the Evi-1 locus expressed transcripts of 4-5 kb while myeloid cell lines without integrations in this locus contained no detectable transcripts.

Based on the Northern analysis, the 58.2 clone appeared to be full length and was therefore sequenced. The sequence contained one large open reading frame following a 5'non-coding region of approximately 500 bp which contained the sequences flanking the viral integration sites. The open reading frame contained a unique sequence which encoded a protein of 120 kd. Comparison of the predicted amino acid sequence with the protein sequence data bank indicated that the protein contained several repeats of the Zinc finger motif. This structure was initially identified in TFIIIA, a frog transcription regulatory factor which controls the transcription of the ribosomal 5S genes during development and has been shown to be responsible for DNA binding activity (Honda, and Roeder, 1980; Pelham, and Brown, 1980; Miller et al.1985). Subsequently a wide variety of transcriptional factors have been shown to contain Zinc fingers (Evans, and Hollenberg, 1988; Berg, 1986). As indicated in figure 4, the Evi-1 locus gene product contains 10 repeats of a 28 amino acid repeat which is characterized by the placement of the histidines, phenylalanine, leucine and cysteines. Seven of the repeats occur in the amino terminus of the gene where there are six contiguous repeats separated from the first repeat by 25 amino acids. Three contiguous repeats are localized in the carboxyl region near a highly acidic domain which shares limited similarity to an acid domain in the c-myc gene and is a common feature of transcriptional regulatory proteins.

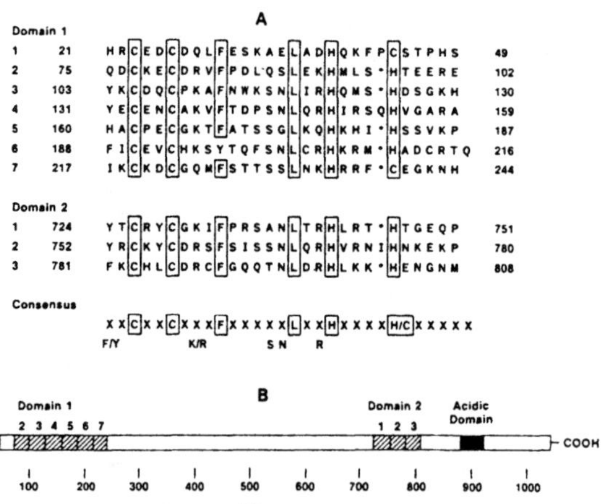

Fig. 4. Structure of the Zinc finger repeats and location within the Evi-1 Gene. The amino acid sequences of the 10 finger repeat regions are shown in A and the consensus sequence is shown at the bottom. The schematic organization of the predicted protein is shown in B. An acidic domain is indicated by the solid boxed area and the finger repeats are indicated by the cross-hatched boxes.

Taken together the results demonstrate that retroviral insertions in the *Evi*-1 locus in IL3-dependent cell lines result in the activation of the expression of a gene encoding a transcriptional regulatory protein containing the Zinc finger DNA binding structure. Viral integrations occur in the 5' region of the gene near 5' non-coding exons and activate transcription by promoter insertion in the examples characterized to date.

CB-1/Fim-3 Common Sites of Integration are Genetically Linked to Evi-1.

To identify additional genes which might be associated with the transformation of IL3-dependent myeloid cells, we have isolated viral integration sites from cell lines lacking rearrangements of known loci. Initially the DA-3 cell line was chosen and 60 genomic clones containing 6 unique integration sites were isolated from a Sau3A partial library. From among the clones containing unique viral integration sites, one clone contained a cellular locus (termed CB-1) which was also rearranged in the DA-34, IL3-dependent cell line and was therefore further characterized.

A restriction map, encompassing approximately 18 kb of the locus, was developed from 3 overlapping genomic clones. In the DA-3 cell line the rearrangement involved a single LTR integrated in the locus whereas in DA-34 cells a more complete provirus was present. Inspection of the *CB*-1 locus restriction map indicated that it was identical to the restriction map of the *Fim*-3 locus, a common integration site for Friend MuLV in a series of myeloid cell lines (Bordereaux et al.1987).

Unique sequence probes from the CB-1/*Fim*-3 locus were used in genetic mapping experiments to determine its chromosomal location. Using interspecific backcrosses, the CB-1/*Fim*-3 locus was mapped to chromosome 3 and was found to be tightly linked to the *Evi*-1 locus such that there were no recombinations detected among 151 mice. To determine whether a possible physical linkage existed between the CB-1/*Fim*-3 locus and the *Evi*-1 locus, additional genomic clones were isolated for the CB-1 locus and the *Evi*-1 locus and restriction maps developed. To date, there is no apparent physical overlap between approximately 70 kb of the CB-1 locus which has been mapped and approximately 40 kb of the *Evi*-1 locus. A potential relationship between the two loci is strongly indicated however by the observation that viral integrations in the CB-1 locus are associated with the expression of transcripts detectable with the probes for the *Evi*-1 gene product (Figure 3). Experiments are currently in progress to further determine the relationship between the two loci.

DISCUSSION

The transformation of hematopoietic cells can alter the requirement of the cells for growth factors, alter the ability of the cells to differentiate or both. A wide variety of studies have examined the effects of oncogenes on growth factor requirements of hematopoietic cells (Carimer, and Samarut, 1986; Cook et al.1985; Pierce et al.1985; Rapp et al.1985). These studies have shown that a number of tyrosine protein kinase containing oncogenes can abrogate the requirements for hematopoietic growth factors. In contrast relatively few studies have addressed the effects of oncogenes on the normal differentiation of hematopoietic cells. In our experience over the past several years, none of the transforming viruses we have examined have had an effect on normal IL3-supported differentiation.

To identify genes which might alter differentiation we have focused our efforts on IL3-dependent cell lines isolated from myeloid leukemias. These cells have normal responses to hematopoietic growth factors but are blocked in there ability to terminally differentiate. For these reasons we have hypothesized that transformation has primarily affected differentiation and thus might allow the identification of a unique set of transforming genes. Among the known oncogenes examined only rearrangements of the c-myb gene have been found in IL3-dependent lines. This was particularly striking because of the myeloid lineage specificity of the transforming activity of the v-myb gene and its speculated role in affecting differentiation. To extend these observations it will be necessary to determine the effect of the expression of a truncated murine c-myb gene on the differentiation of IL3-dependent cells.

In addition to the rearrangement of the c-myb gene, NFS-60 cells contain a viral integration in the Evi-1 locus. Consequently it has not been possible to determine whether both genes have affected the ability of the cells to differentiate or whether one of the genes has affected the cells in an undefined manner. Other cell lines containing myb gene rearrangements have a more mature myeloid lineage phenotypes while the NFS-60 cell line has an immature phenotype. Thus it is possible that a hematopoietic stem cell initially contained only the myb gene rearrangement and the cells were altered in differentiation but not sufficient for malignant transformation. Subsequently retroviral activation of the Evi-1 locus occurred and caused further transformation.

A number of the IL3-dependent lines contain viral insertions in either the Evi-1 locus or the CB-1/Fim-3 locus resulting in the expression of a protein with structural similarities to transcriptional regulatory proteins. Although the physical linkage has not been established, these loci are closely linked genetically. More strikingly however, cell lines containing viral integrations in the CB-1/Fim-3 locus and cell lines with viral integrations in the CB-1/Fim-3 locus express the Evi-1 gene. Experiments are currently in progress to determine the physical linkage between these loci and to define the mechanism of activation of expression of the Evi-1 gene in cells containing viral integrations in the CB-1/Fim-3 locus.

Among the cell lines examined in these studies six out of eight contained viral integrations in the Evi-1/CB-1/Fim-3 loci. Among all the lines available, integrations in these loci occur in approximately 15% of the cells. Among Friend MuLV cell lines, approximately 42% contained viral integrations in the Fim-3 locus. Taken together the data suggest that activation of the expression of the Evi-1 gene is the most frequent event associated with myeloid lineage transformation. Also of interest is the observation that activation of the Evi-1 gene has been uniquely associated with myeloid transformation in the models that have been examined. This suggests that the altered expression of the Evi-1 gene may be specific for myeloid lineage transformation. Irrespective it will now be important to examine a variety of transformed cell types for rearrangements and activation of the expression of the Evi-1 gene.

The frequency with which activation of the Evi-1 gene occurs in murine myeloid leukemias suggests that it might also be important in human leukemias. To address this question we have mapped the Evi-1 gene to the long arm of human chromosome 3 at band q25.1 (Morishita, Sacchi, Valentine and Ihle, unpublished data). This region has been shown to be involved in translocations and inversions in myelodysplastic disease as well as in myeloid leukemias (Akahoshi et al.1987; Bernstein et al.1986; Bitter et al.1985; Rubin et al.1987; Shimazaki et al.1986). Experiments are currently in progress to determine whether these translocations involved the Evi-1 locus.

ACKNOWLEDGEMENT

Research sponsored by the National Cancer Institute, DHHS, under contract No. NO1-CO-74101 with Bionetics Research Inc. The contents of this publication do not necessarily reflect the views or policies of the Department of Health and Human Services, nor does mention of trade names, commercial products, or organizations imply endorsement by the U.S. Government. We would like to thank Marlene R. Jacks for her help in preparing the manuscript.

REFERENCES

Akahoshi M, Oshimi K, Mizoguchi H, Okada M, Enomoto Y, Watanabe Y (1987) Myeloproliferative disorders terminating in acute megakaryoblastic leukemia with chromosome 3q26 abnormality. Cancer 60: 2654-2661

Berg J. (1986). Potential metal-binding domains in nucleic acid binding proteins. Science 232: 485-487

Bernstein R, Bagg A, Pinto M, Lewis D, Mendelow B (1986) Chromosome 3q21 abnormalities associated with hyperactive thrombopoiesis in acute blastic transformation of chronic myeloid leukemia. Blood 68: 652-657

Beug HM, Hayman J, Graf T (1982) Myeloblasts transformed by the avian acute leukemia virus E26 are hormone-dependent for growth and for expression of a putative myb-containing protein. EMBO J 1: 1063-1073

Bitter MA, Neilly ME, LeBeau MM, Pearson MG, Rowley JD (1985) Rearrangements of chromosome 3 involving bands 3q21 and 3q26 are associated with normal or elevated platelet counts in acute nonlymphocytic leukemia. Blood 66: 1362-1370

Bordereaux D, Fichelson S, Sola B, Tambourin PE, Gisselbrecht S (1987) Frequent involvement of the fim-3 region in Friend murine leukemia virus-induced mouse myeloblastic leukemias. J Virol 61: 4043-4045

Carimer JF, Samarut J (1986) Chicken myeloid cells infected by retroviruses carrying the v-fps oncogene do not require exogenous growth factors to differentiate in vitro. Cell 44: 159-165

Cook WD, Metcalf D, Nicola NA, Burgess AW, Walker F (1985) Malignant transformation of a growth factor-dependent myeloid cell line by

Abelson virus without evidence of an autocrine mechanism. Cell 41: 677-683

Evans RM, Hollenberg SM (1988) Zinc fingers: gilt by association minireview. Cell 52: 1-3

Holmes KL, Palaszynski E, Fredrickson TN, Morse HC 3d, Ihle JN (1985) Correlation of cell-surface phenotype with the establishment of interleukin 3-dependent cell lines from wild-mouse murine leukemia virus-induced neoplasms. Proc Natl Acad Sci USA 82: 6687-6691

Honda BM, Roeder RG (1980) Association of a 5S gene transcription factor with 5S RNA and altered levels of the factor during cell differentiation. Cell 22: 19203-126

Ihle JN, Rein A, Mural R (1984) Immunological and virological mechanisms in retrovirus induced murine leukemogenesis. In: Klein G (ed) Advances in Viral Oncology, Vol 4. Raven Press, New York, pp 95-137

Ihle JN, Weinstein Y (1986) Immunological regulation of hematopoietic/lymphoid stem cell differentiation by interleukin 3. Adv Immunol 39: 1-50

Ihle JN (1988) The molecular and cellular biology of interleukin-3. In: Cruse JM, Lewis RE Jr (eds) The Year in Immunology. Karger, New York, in press

Joyner A, Keller G, Phillips RA, Bernstein A (1983) Retrovirus transfer of a bacterial gene into mouse haematopoietic progenitor cells. Nature 305: 556-558

Keller G, Paige C, Gilboa E, Wagner EF (1985) Expression of a foreign gene in myeloid and lymphoid cells derived from multipotent haematopoietic precursors. Nature 318: 149-154

Klempnauer KH, Gonda T, Bishop JM (1982) Nucleotide sequence of the retroviral leukemia gene v-myb and its cellular progenitor c-myb: the architecture of a transduced oncogene. Cell 31: 453-463

Klempnauer KH, Ramsay G, Bishop JM, Moscovici MG, Moscovici C, McGrath JP, Levinson AD (1983) The product of the retroviral transforming gene v-myb is a truncated version of the protein encoded by the cellular oncogene c-myb. Cell 33: 345-355

Lee JC, Ihle JN (1981) Increased responses to lymphokines are correlated with preleukemia in mice inoculated with Moloney leukemia virus. Proc Natl Acad Sci USA 78: 7712-7716

Lee JC, Horak I, Ihle JN (1981a) Mechanisms in T-cell leukemogenesis. II. T-cell responses of preleukemic BALB/c mice to Moloney leukemia virus antigens. J Immunol 126: 715-722

Lee JC, Ihle JN (1981b) Chronic immune stimulation is required for Moloney leukemia virus-induced lymphomas. Nature 289: 407-409

Lemischka IR, Raulet DH, Mulligan RC (1986) Developmental potential and dynamic behavior of hematopoietic stem cells. Cell 45: 917-927

Miller J, McLachlan AD, Klug A (1985) Repetitive zinc-binding domains in the protein transcription factor IIIA from Xenopus oocytes. EMBO J 4: 1609-1614

Morishita K, Parker DS, Mucenski ML, Jenkins NA, Copeland NG, Ihle JN (1988) Retroviral activation of a novel gene encoding a zinc finger protein in IL-3-dependent myeloid leukemia cell lines. Cell 54: in press

Moscovici MG, Jurdic P, Samarut J, Gazzolo L, Mura CV, Moscovici C (1983) Characterization of the hemopoietic target cells for the avian leukemia virus E26. Virology 129: 65-78

Mucenski ML, Taylor BA, Ihle JN, Hartley JW, Morse HC 3d, Jenkins NA, Copeland NG (1988) Identification of a common ecotropic viral integration site, Evi-1, in the DNA of AKXD murine myeloid tumors. Mol Cell Biol 8: 301-308

Pelham HR, Brown DD (1980) A specific transcription factor that can bind either the 5S RNA gene or 5S RNA. Proc Natl Acad Sci USA 77: 4170-4174

Pierce JH, Di Fiore PP, Aaronson SA, Potter M, Pumphrey J, Scott A, Ihle JN (1985) Neoplastic transformation of mast cells by Abelson-MuLV: abrogation of IL-3 dependence by a nonautocrine mechanism. Cell 41: 685-693

Rapp UR, Cleveland JL, Brightman K, Scott A, Ihle JN (1985) Abrogation of IL-3 and IL-2 dependence by recombinant murine retroviruses expressing v-myc oncogenes. Nature 317: 434-438

Rubin CM, Larson RA, Bitter MA, Carrino JJ, LeBeau MM, Diaz MO, Rowley JD (1987) Association of a chromosomal 3:21 translocation with the blast phase of chronic myelogenous leukemia. Blood 70: 1338-1342

Shimazaki C, Fujita N, Nakanishi S, Nishio A, Haruyama H, Nakagawa M, Ijichi H, Nishida K, Misawa S (1986) Inversion of chromosome 3 in a case of chronic myelogenous leukemia with abnormal thrombopoiesis. Cancer Genet Cytogenet 20: 121-127

Weinstein Y, Ihle JN, Lavu S, Reddy EP (1986) Truncation of the c-myb gene by a retroviral integration in an interleukin-3 dependent myeloid leukemia cell line. Proc Natl Acad Sci USA 83: 5010-5014

Weinstein Y, Cleveland JL, Askew DS, Rapp UR, Ihle JN (1987) Insertion and truncation of c-myb by MuLV in a myeloid cell line derived from cultures of normal hematopoietic cells. J Virol 61: 2339-2343

Williams DA, Lemischka IR, Nathans DG, Mulligan RC (1984) Introduction of new genetic material into pluripotent haematopoietic stem cells of the mouse. Nature 310: 476-480

Alternate Forms of *MYB:* Consequences of Virus Insertion in Myeloid Tumorigenesis and Alternative Splicing in Normal Development

Grace L.C. Shen-Ong

Laboratory of Genetics, National Cancer Institute, Bethesda, MD 20892

INTRODUCTION

Nearly half of the proto-oncogenes were first identified in the genome of highly oncogenic avian and mammalian retroviruses (for review, see Bishop 1985). Several of these oncogenes appear to selectively transform cells of a particular lineage of differentiation. Studies on the v-myb containing avian myeloblastosis virus (AMV) and E-26 leukemia virus suggest that the viral oncogene v-myb is closely associated with myeloid tumorigenesis (for review, see Graf 1988). The transduction that gave rise to v-myb truncated the protooncogene c-myb at both of its ends. It is conceivable that myb may have multiple functions carried out by different structural domains. Removal of any of these domains may abolish either some function(s) performed by myb or its ability to be regulated by interaction with other cellular proteins. In order to understand the role of myb in normal and tumor development of myeloid cells, it is important to identify the various forms of myb in different cell types.

ALTERNATE FORMS OF MYB IN MYELOID TUMORIGENESIS

5' Disruption of MYB by Virus Insertion in Murine Myeloid Tumors

A unique group of tumors, termed Abelson virus-induced plasmacytoid lymphosarcomas (ABPLs), had been shown to carry a disrupted allele of the c-myb locus due to the insertion of the Moloney murine leukemia virus (M-MuLV), the helper component of the Abelson virus complex (Shen-Ong et al 1984). Subsequent cellular and molecular studies have demonstrated that the tumor cells belong to the myelomonocytic lineage, and the tumors have thus been renamed as myelogenous leukemias (ABMLs) (Shen-Ong et al 1987). Recent tumor induction experiments showed that M-MuLV alone is sufficient to induce ABML-like tumors in adult Balb/c mice provided that the mice had been pristane-primed (Shen-Ong and Wolff 1987). The M-MuLV induced tumors (termed MMLs) resembled ABMLs both genotypically with respect to clonal c-myb activation by M-MuLV insertion, and phenotypically in many aspects.

Current Topics in Microbiology and Immunology, Vol. 149

Fig. 1 shows that the M-MuLV had clonally inserted within a 3.0-kbp span of the 5'-end of the c-myb gene in all seven MMLs examined. Similar results were obtained for six different ABMLs (Shen-Ong et al. 1986).

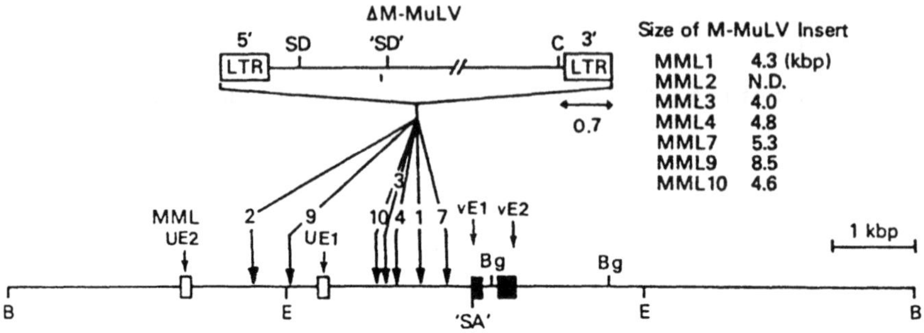

Fig. 1. Map of the c-myb genetic region that is altered by the insertion of an M-MuLV component. The size of the deleted M-MuLV insert in the rearranged fragment (right panel) was estimated by determining the increase in size of the normal 4.2-kbp EcoRI fragment found in each MML. Open and solid boxes indicate the four myb coding exons from left to right as the upstream 5' UE2 and UE1 exons, which are absent in the gag-myb mRNAs, and the first two vE1 and vE2 exons with v-myb homology.

The MYB Locus in the Target Cells for M-MuLV Induced Myeloid Tumors is Probably Transcriptionally Active

The clustering of the viral integrations within the myb locus may indicate the presence of a hot spot for integration. It has been shown that MMLs were obtained only when pristane-primed mice were intravenously (i.v.) injected but not when intraperitoneally (i.p.) injected (Wolff et al 1988), suggesting that a higher proportion of cells capable of being transformed by M-MuLV are located in tissues outside of the peritoneal cavity. The relative levels of c-myb expression in the different tissues of pristane-primed mice 3 weeks after M-MuLV infection are determined by RNase mapping studies (Fig.2). No myb expression is found in the ascitic cells (predominantly mature myeloid cells) obtained from the peritoneal cavity even upon prolonged exposure of the gel, whereas variable levels of c-myb expression are found in cells obtained from the thymus, bone marrow and to a much lesser extent the spleen. Taken together, it is likely that the cells that are capable of being transformed by M-MuLV carry transcriptionally active myb allele(s).

Earlier studies showed a reduction in the level of c-myb expression in hematopoietic cells induced to differentiate (Westin et al 1982), suggesting that the myb oncogene may induce both cell proliferation and a block of differentiation. Myb expression from the virus-disrupted allele in the MML10 clonal cell line remains high (Fig.2) even though the cells became phenotypically more mature after establishment and passaging in vitro. Presumably, this aberrant myb expression maintains the tumor cells in their proliferative state.

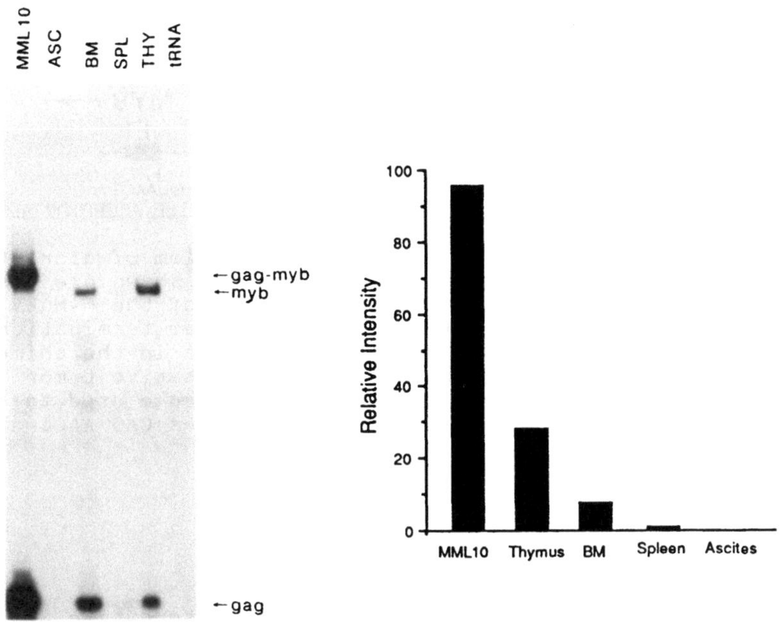

Fig. 2. Relative levels of myb expression in different tissues. RNase protection studies (left) of myb transcript from MML10 tumor cells and cells obtained from the ascites (ASC, 20μg), bone marrow (BM, 30μg), spleen (SPL, 20μg) and thymus (THY, 15μg) of pristane-primed mice 3 weeks after M-MuLV infection via intravenous injection. The ^{32}P-labeled antisense transcript probe was obtained from a gag-myb chimeric cDNA clone, and contains 160 bases of gag sequences (starting at the PvuII site within gag p30) linked via splicing to 342 bases of myb vE1 to vE3 sequences (ending at the EcoRI site within vE3 exon). The experiment was performed as previously described (Shen-Ong, 1987). The intensity of the various protected myb hybrids were measured by densitometer scanning and corrected for the amount of total RNA used in each protection sample. The relative intensity of myb expression in different tissues based on these measurements was shown (right).

Truncation of 5'Coding Sequences of MYB in ABMLs and MMLs

cDNA cloning and S1 mapping analyses revealed that the consistent finding of proviral integration within the 5'-end of the c-myb gene in all the ABMLs and MMLs examined led to transcription from the inserted M-MuLV promoter a chimeric viral gag-myb species that lacks the three normal 5'-most c-myb coding exons (UE3, UE2 and UE1, Fig. 3, Shen-Ong et al 1986, Shen-Ong & Wolff 1987). Since the open reading frames of the gag and myb sequences in the chimeric transcripts are out of frame with each other, an internal translational start site within the gag p30 sequences is probably used to generate a tumor-specific myb gene product that is truncated in the N-terminus. The extents of 5' truncation as a result of either provirus insertion in murine tumors or myb transduction in two different avian retroviruses are the same suggests that this structural alteration is important in the activation of the c-myb gene in tumor development.

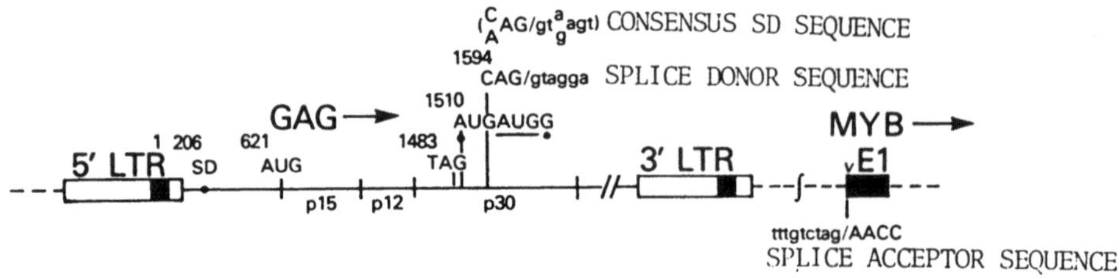

Fig. 3. Schematic diagram illustrating the mechanism of disruption of the c-myb locus in ABMLs and MMLs. The numbers shown are positions of the following viral sequences: 1, the cap site of the M-MuLV; 206, the viral splice donor sequence (SD); 1483, upstream termination codon in the same reading frame as the myb sequence in the chimeric gag-myb transcripts; 1510, sequences around the putative tumor myb start codon; 1594, the novel splice donor sequence used to generate the chimeric RNA resulting in the sequences CAG/AACC at the splice junction.

ALTERNATE FORMS OF MYB IN NORMAL CELLS

In Frame Additional Internal Exon Resulted from Alternative Splicing in MYB Transcripts Expressed from the Normal and Provirus-activated MYB Gene in Both Normal and Tumor Cells

An alternative splicing event towards the 3' side of the myb gene (in the vicinity where the transduced v-myb genes in two different avian retroviruses end) has recently been found in several ABMLs, and was suggested to be induced by the 5'-M-MuLV insertion, thus playing a crucial role in the activation of the myb gene (Rosson and Reddy 1987). However, RNA blot and RNase mapping analyses show that a significant portion (~10%) of all myb transcripts examined, whether in normal or in clonal tumor cells contain an in frame additional 363-bp internal exon (termed E6A) as the result of the same splicing event as reported for ABMLs (Shen-Ong 1987). Thus a consistent and major determinant in the generation of M-MuLV-induced myeloid tumors is the 5' alteration of the c-myb product by insertional mutagenesis. Since myb is thought to be involved in induction of cell proliferation, block of differentiation and even reversal of differention, the additional exon found in a minor population of normal c-myb transcripts may constitute a separate domain that is required for a particular biologic function.

DETECTION OF THE PUTATIVE 5'-TRUNCATED AND E6A-CONTAINING MYB PROTEINS IN CELLS

The nucleotide sequences of the tumor myb cDNA clone define a potential coding domain of 592 amino acids residues for the product of tumor-specific *myb* (Shen-Ong et al 1986). Using antibodies directed against a bacterial fusion protein that contains the domain encoded by the highly conserved 5' one-third of the v-*myb* oncogene of AMV (a generous gift from J. Lipsick, Boyle et al 1986), we have identified a $p70^{(tu\text{-}myb)}$ in ABML cells by immunoprecipitation studies (Fig. 4, in collaboration with Robert Eisenman). The tumor-specific *myb* product which is truncated in the N-terminus is smaller than the normal $p75^{(c\text{-}myb)}$ that contains 636 amino acid residues. We have also identified a $p80^{(tu\text{-}myb)}$ protein in the ABML cells and a $p85^{(c\text{-}myb)}$ protein in cells that carry the normal c-*myb* locus (Fig.4). These two larger forms of *myb* are probably encoded by the E6A-containing *myb* transcripts. None of the *myb* products is detected by antisera that had been preincubated with excess antigen (data not shown). Hence multiple forms of *myb* are present in different cell types.

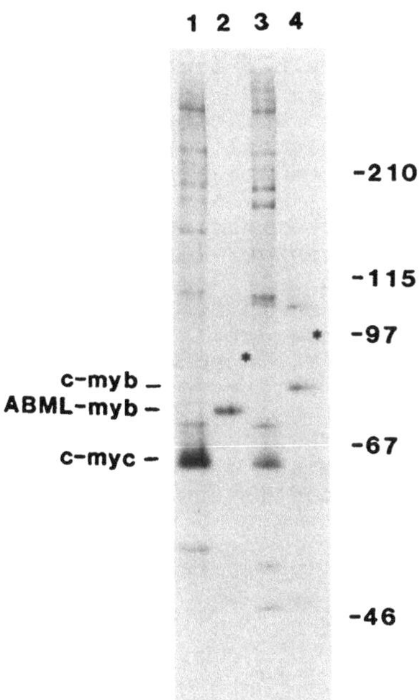

Fig. 4. Identification of the ABML truncated *myb* protein by immunoprecipitation analysis. Extracts of $[^{35}S]$ methionine-labeled AMBL4.6 cells with 5'-truncated *myb* locus (lane 1,2) and 70Z cells with normal c-*myb* locus (lane 3,4) were immunoprecipitated with rabbit antiserum raised against *myc* peptides (lane 1,3) or bacterially expressed v-*myb* protein (lane 2,4). Immunoprecipi tated proteins were electrophoresed in SDS-polyacrylamide gels and visualized by autoradiography. Asterisks marked the putative E6A containing proteins. Sizes are indicated in kilodaltons.

FUTURE PROSPECTS

The studies presented here demonstrate that both the levels of *myb* expression and the structure of the *myb* gene product are altered by insertional mutagenesis in myeloid tumors. More studies will be required in order to determine if the deregulation of *myb*, or the structural alteration, or both is important in myeloid tumorigenesis. The identification of E6A-containing *myb* products in cells that carry either virus-disrupted *myb* or normal c-*myb* gene shows that *myb* belongs to the class of proteins that possess structural diversity. Exploring the regulation of expression and biochemical properties of the different forms of *myb* during normal and tumor development of myeloid cells should be important in the elucidation of the role of *myb* in these processes.

REFERENCES

Bishop JM (1985) Viral oncogenes. Cell 42:23-38
Boyle WJ, Lipsick JS, Baluda MA (1986) Antibodies to the evolutionarily conserved amino-terminal region of the v-myb encoded protein detect the c-myb protein in widely divergent metazoan species. Proc Natl Acad Sci USA 83:4685-4689.
Graf T (1988) Leukemia as a multistep process: Studies with avian retroviruses containing two oncogenes. Leukemia 2:127-131
Rosson D, Dugan D, Reddy EP (1987) Aberrant splicing events that are induced by proviral integration: Implications for myb oncogene activation. Proc Natl Acad Sci USA 84:3171-3175
Shen-Ong GLC, Potter M, Mushinski JF, Lavu S, Reddy EP (1984) Activation of the c-myb locus by viral insertional mutagenesis in plasmacytoid lymphosarcomas. Science 226:1077-1080
Shen-Ong GLC, Morse III HC, Potter M, Mushinski JF (1986) Two modes of c-myb activation in virus-induced mouse myeloid tumors. Mol Cell Biol 6:380-392
Shen-Ong GLC, Holmes KL, Morse III HC (1987) Phorbol ester-induced growth arrest of murine myelomonocytic leukemia cells with virus-disrupted myb locus is not accompanied by decreased myc and myb expression. Proc Natl Acad Sci USA 84:199-203
Shen-Ong GLC, Wolff L (1987) Moloney murine leukemia virus-induced myeloid tumors in adult BALB/c mice: requirement of c-myb activation but lack of v-abl involvement. J Virol 61:3721-3725
Shen-Ong GLC (1987) Alternative internal splicing in c-myb RNAs occurs commonly in normal and tumor cells. EMBO J 6:4035-4039
Westin EH, Gallo RC, Arya SK, Souza LM, Baluda MA, Aaronson SA, Wong-Staal, F (1982) Differential expression of the amv gene in human hematopoietic cells. Proc Natl Acad Sci USA 79:2194-2198
Wolff L, Mushinski JF, Shen-Ong GLC, Morse III HC (1988) A chronic inflammatory response: Its role in supporting the development of c-myb and c-myc related promonocytic and monocytic tumors in BALB/c mice. J Immunol 141:681-689

IV. Myeloid Leukemogensis Induced by Acute Transforming Virus Constructs in In Vitro and In Vivo Model Systems

Retrovirus-Induced Tumors Whose Development is Facilitated by a Chronic Immune Response: A Comparison of Two Tumors Committed to the Monocytic Lineage

Linda Wolff and Kathryn Nason-Burchenal

Laboratory of Genetics, National Cancer Institute, National Institutes of Health, Bethesda, Maryland

INTRODUCTION

An active immune response can under certain circumstances facilitate induction of neoplasms (Schwartz and Beldotti 1965; Gleichmann et al, 1984; Potter 1986; Baumbach et al 1986; Potter et al 1987; Wolff et al 1986 ; Wolff et al 1988). Our studies, in particular, have shown that a chronic inflammatory granuloma in the peritoneal cavity can promote the rapid induction of myeloid tumors by retroviruses (Wolff et al 1986; Wolff et al 1988). Two myeloid tumors that arose in the peritoneal cavity of pristane-primed BALB/cAnPt mice were (a) the McML, mature monocyte-macrophage tumors induced by retroviral constructs containing exons 2 and 3 of the c-myc cDNA and (b) the MML, promonocytic tumors induced by Moloney murine leukemia virus (M-MuLV).

MECHANISMS OF DISEASE INDUCTION

Figure 1 depicts the mechanisms by which we propose that these two neoplasms develop. Prior to the inoculation of the above mentioned retroviruses, a chronic inflammatory response is established by injection of pristane into the peritoneal cavity. This causes an overall stimulation of the myeloid compartment and results in an observed influx of mature macrophages and granulocytes and perhaps immature myeloid cells as well. As shown in part A of Figure 1, when retrovirus constructs containing the c-myc gene in conjunction with Moloney MuLV (which provides helper virus functions) are inoculated intraperitoneally they infect monocytic cells in the peritoneal cavity and transform them. The McML tumors become evident in ascites smears at 2 to 3 months at which time they appear morphologically as mature macrophage cells. It is not clear, however, if these cells were infected prior to their becoming fully differentiated cells or if they become infected and immortalized while in their final stage of development. Mice that do not receive pristane do not develop tumors which suggests that the peritoneal cavity provides a specialized growth environment for rapid proliferation of these cells. In addition, this environment may promote a necessary secondary oncogenic event that increases the malignant potential of the cells.

The other myeloid tumor (MML) that has a more immature monocytic cell phenotype is induced by intravenous (i.v.) inoculation of Moloney MuLV virus by itself. Intravenous injection is apparently critical and suggests that the cells that ultimately become transformed are infected early on by the virus within organs that are readily

Current Topics in Microbiology and Immunology, Vol. 149

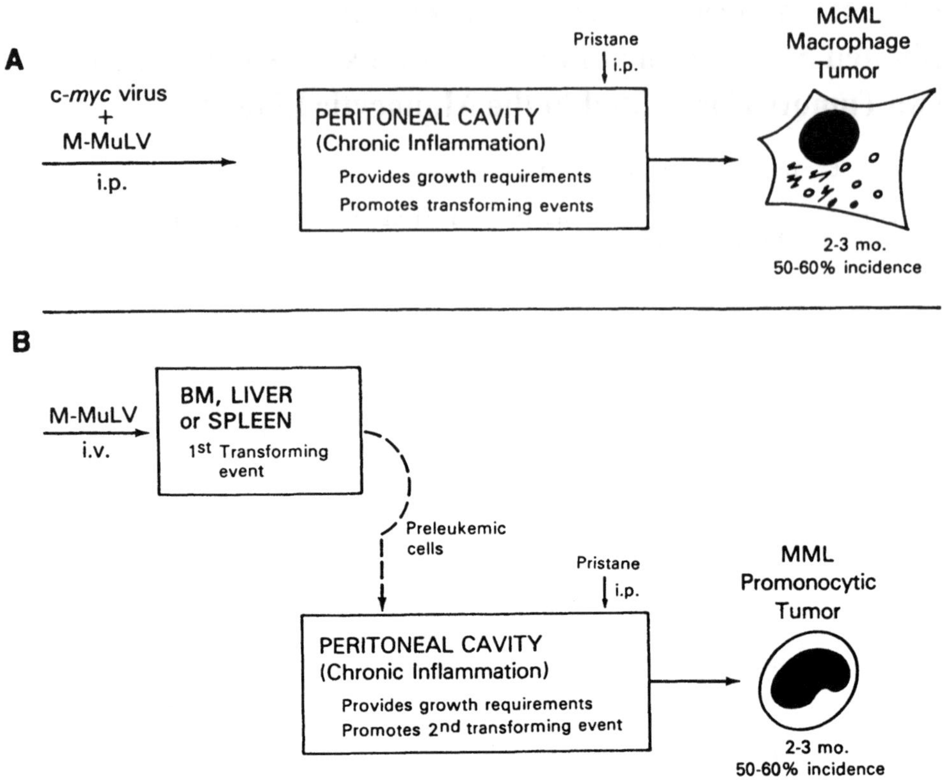

Fig. 1. Proposed mechanisms for development of two myeloid tumors induced by retroviruses. A) Development of mature monocyte-macrophage tumors by c-myc containing retrovirus vectors B) Development of promonocytic tumors by Moloney MuLV.

accessible by i.v. injection. We have found, as shown in Table 1,that pristane primed mice have an increased number of GM-CSF responsive myeloid precursor cells (CFU-C) in their spleens and livers when compared to aged matched nonprimed controls. Whether this increase in precursor cells contributes to the rapid and reproducible induction of disease remains to be determined. In any case, it is likely that preleukemic cells infected with Moloney MuLV migrate into the peritoneal cavity where the conditions of the inflammatory response provide a growth advantage and perhaps promotion of a transforming event. It has been shown that all the BALB/cAnPt promonocytic neoplasms so far examined have virus integrated in the 5'end of the c-myb locus (Shen-Ong and Wolff 1987). It is possible that other oncogene activations may also occur as a result of viral integration, mutation, or chromosomal rearrangement.

We have recently tested the susceptibility of three other strains of mice, BALB/cJax, DBA/2, and C57BL/6, that were shown to be resistent to pristane-dependent plasmacytoma induction (Potter 1984). As shown in Table 2, BALBc/Jax mice were just as susceptible to induction of tumors by Moloney MuLV as BALB/cAnPt mice from Exp.II that were inoculated at the same time and with the same virus stocks. DBA/2 mice were also susceptible and it was found that DBA/2 mice had a higher incidence of disease but a slightly longer latency. DNAs from 2 BALB/cJax tumors and 7 DBA/2 tumors were examined for c-myb gene rearrangements and altered genes were found in all but one of the DBA/2 tumors (data not shown) suggesting that these promonocytic tumors were analogous to those previously described in BALB/c AnPt mice. BALB/cJax and DBA/2 mice do not develop myeloid tumors as a result of pristane priming alone (our own data). C57BL/6 mice, unlike the other strains, were essentially resistant to the disease; only one mouse developed a tumor 176 days post virus inoculation which appeared morphologically to have a mature macrophage phenotype and it was not possible to demonstrate a rearrangement of the c-myb locus in the DNA from this tumor.

TABLE I. Quantitative Comparison of Committed Myeloid Precursor Cells in Hematopoietic Organs of Pristane-Primed and Unprimed mice.[1]

Exp. No.	Pristane	Days post Pristane[2]	Bone Marrow CFC[3]	Bone Marrow P+/P-[4]	Spleen CFC	Spleen P+/P-	Liver CFC	Liver P+/P-
1	-		440		0		1.5	
1	+	23	210	<1	32	>32[5]	8.0	5.3
2	-		280		2.5		0.5	
2	+	25	195	<1	7.0	2.8	7.0	14
3	-		365		3.5		0	
3	+	29	662	1.8	27	7.7	9.5	>9.5
4	-		445		0		0.5	
4	+	30	440	<1.0	41	>41	16.0	8.0
5	-		170		3.0		0.5	
5	+	35	250	1.5	26	8.7	9.5	19
6	-		265		1.0		0	
6	+	37	275	1.0	7.5	7.5	3.5	>3.5
7	-		190		0		0	
7	+	38	200	1.1	10	>10	0.5	>0.5

[1]The clonigenic assay for quantitating myeloid colony-forming cells (CFC) was a modification of that of Metcalf (1984). The cells were cultured using 0.35% Seaplaque agarose (Rockland, ME) in RPMI 1640 supplemented with 20% fetal calf serum. Recombinant mouse GM-CSF from Genzyme (Boston, MA) used at a concentration of 50u/ml.

[2]Mice received 0.5ml pristane intraperitoneally.

[3]CFC per 5×10^5 cells. These numbers are the average count of duplicate plates.

[4]CFC in pristane primed mouse divided by CFC in unprimed mouse in the same experiment

[5]Limit of detection for spleen and liver cells was 1 per 5×10^5 cells.

Moloney MuLV typically causes T cell lymphomas in both primed and unprimed mice, but with a longer average latency than the promonocytic tumors. Since development of the lymphoid disease has been shown to be associated with the formation of recombinant mink cell focus-forming (MCF) viruses we questioned whether MCF viruses might play a role in the development of the promonocytic tumors (MML). To answer this question MML established tumor cell lines were examined for the presence of MCF virus-specific envelope proteins. Cells were pulse-labeled with ^{35}S-methionine, and extracted proteins were immune precipitated with MCF specific antiserum and separated on polyacrylamide gels. Two of the three lines tested did not express proteins

Table II. Induction of Myeloid Tumors by M-MuLV In Different Strains of Mice

			Myeloid tumors		Lymphomas	
Strain	Virus[1]	Pristane[2]	Incidence	Latency[3]	Incidence	Latency
BALB/cAnPt Exp. I	+	+	14/26(54%)[4]	53-102(76)	2/26(8%)	102,113
	-	+	0/15(0%)	N.A.	0/15(0%)	N.A.
	+	-	0/14(0%)	N.A.	2/13(15%)	106,113
BALB/cAnPt Exp. II	+	+	6/13(46%)	85-112(106)	4/13(30%)	90-141(110)
BALB/cJax	+	+	9/21(43%)	85-125(103)	5/21(23%)	92-174(135)
DBA/2	+	+	9/13(69%)	96-168(118)	1/13(8%)	168
C57BL/6	+	+	1/15(7%)	176	0/15(0%)	N.A.

[1]Virus preparations contained >10^6 XC plaque-forming virus particles per ml. One half of an ml was injected into the tail vein of each mouse.
[2]Mice received 0.5 ml pristane (2,6,10,14-tetramethylpentadecane) intraperitoneally 3 wks prior to virus inoculation.
[3]Range in days with average range in parenthesis
[4]Terminated at 120 d. Remaining groups terminated at 6 mo.

that were precipitable with MCF-specific antiserum, suggesting that MCF viruses were not required for the evolution of these tumors. We also questioned whether Moloney MuLV was specifically required for tumor formation or whether other replication competent retroviruses would be equally capable of initiating the MML disease in pristane-primed mice. When other ecotropic mouse leukemia viruses which are closely related to Moloney MuLV were inoculated into primed BALB/c mice it was found that they were unable to induce tumors analogous to the MML. Retroviruses that were unable to cause disease were the Friend MuLV, a naturally occurring, highly homologous virus, and Mo-MuLV^{sup}, Moloney MuLV which was modified by Reik and colleagues (Reik, Weiher, and Jaenisch 1985) by insertion of the sup^{F} gene into the long terminal repeat region. The latter virus stocks were not defective for replication in vitro since they contained equivalent or greater

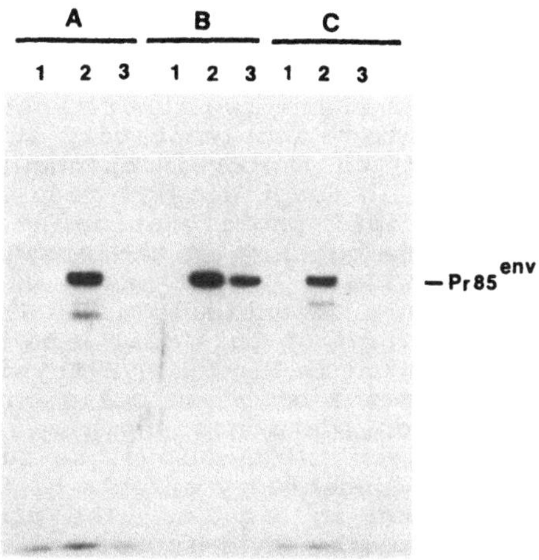

Fig. 2. Immunoprecipitation of retroviral envelope proteins using ecotropic-specific and MCF-specific antiserum. ^{35}S-methionine labeled extracts of WIIB 4-7 (A) WIIB 4-9 (B) and WIIB 4-10 (C) promonocytic tumor cell lines were immunoprecipitated with normal goat serum (1), goat anti-Rauscher MuLV gp70 (recognizes ecotropic and MCF specificities) (2) and MCF gp70 specific antiserum (3).

titers than the Moloney MuLV stocks utilized for the experiments presented in Table II. Furthermore, the Mo-MuLV^{sup} induced lymphoid neoplasms in 2 out of 13 mice (15%). These studies suggest that Moloney-MuLV contains regions that are unique and very specific for induction of MML tumors.

COMPARISON OF THE BIOLOGICAL PROPERTIES OF McML AND MML TUMORS

Initially it was observed that the c-myc virus induced tumors (McML) and the Moloney MuLV induced tumors (MML) were quite different morphologically regardless of the fact that they had similar antigenic markers such as Mac-1, Mac-2 and Fc receptors. For example, the McML cells had a mature phenotype with a high cytoplasmic-to-nuclear ratio, numerous cytoplasmic vacuoles and inclusions and ruffled cellular membranes, whereas the MML cells appeared immature having small cytoplasmic-to-nuclear ratios, smooth membranes and often kidney shaped nuclei (Wolff et al 1986; Wolff et al 1988). The fact that MML cells had weak expression of the Ia antigen on the cell surface compared to the McML also indicated that they were more immature. In an attempt to characterize the cells more fully, they were examined for a number of phenotypic and functional characteristics typical of myeloid cells. The results of the phenotypic and functional studies showed that both tumor types were negative for myeloperoxidase staining but positive for nonspecific esterase staining, lysozyme production and phagocytosis, indicating that both tumor cell types are committed to the monocytic lineage (for details see Wolff et al 1988).

A summary of these characteristics as well as other properties we have analyzed more recently are presented in Table III.

Recently it was discovered that the two tumor types differed in their responses to growth stimulatory and inhibitory substances. The McML cells require no adaptation to factor-independent growth in tissue culture, whereas the MML cells adapt slowly, requiring a lag phase of limited growth prior to rapid proliferation. The latter cells, however, can be adapted more quickly in the presence of recombinant GM-CSF, and one cell line (WIIB 4-9) that has been grown continuously in its presence is now essentially GM-CSF- dependent for proliferation. The growth curve of this cell line in the presence and absence of rGM-CSF is presented in Fig. 3. [^{3}H]thymidine uptake assays also demonstrate the dependence of these cells on growth factor for stimulation of proliferation (data not shown). Another difference that has been observed between the two in vitro tumor cell lines is their response to the growth inhibitory effects of transforming growth factor-beta (TGFβ), as shown in Fig. 4. The proliferation of MML cells is completely inhibited by this factor, whereas proliferation of McML cells is only slightly affected. Two other cell lines, a murine erythroleukemia cell line and a plasmacytoma cell line,

TABLE III. Comparison of c-myc-and c-myb-related Tumors Induced in Pristane-primed Mice

Properties	McML (c-myc virus)	MML (M-MuLV)
Similar		
Cell surface markers		
Mac-1,Mac-2,	+	+
Fc-receptor	+	+
Nonspecific esterase	+	+
Lysozyme	+	+
Phagocytosis	+	+
Myeloperoxidase	-	-
Different		
Morphology	mature (monocyte/macrophage)	immature (promonocyte)
Adaptation to culture without CSF	immediate adaptation	slow adaptation
Proliferation in response to CSF	rapid growth in absense	response to GM-CSF
TGFβ sensitivity	+	+++
Induction inhibitable by indomethacin	0%	100%

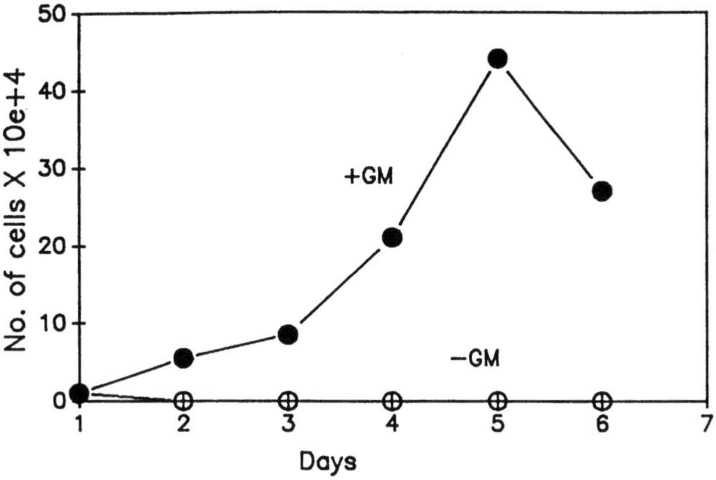

Fig.3. Growth curve of promonocytic tumor cell line, WIIB 4-9, in the presence of rGM-CSF. Cells were seeded on day 1 at a concentration of 1 x 10^5 cells per ml in the presence of 10u/ml rGM-CSF (Genzyme). Cell counts were determined daily up to day 6.

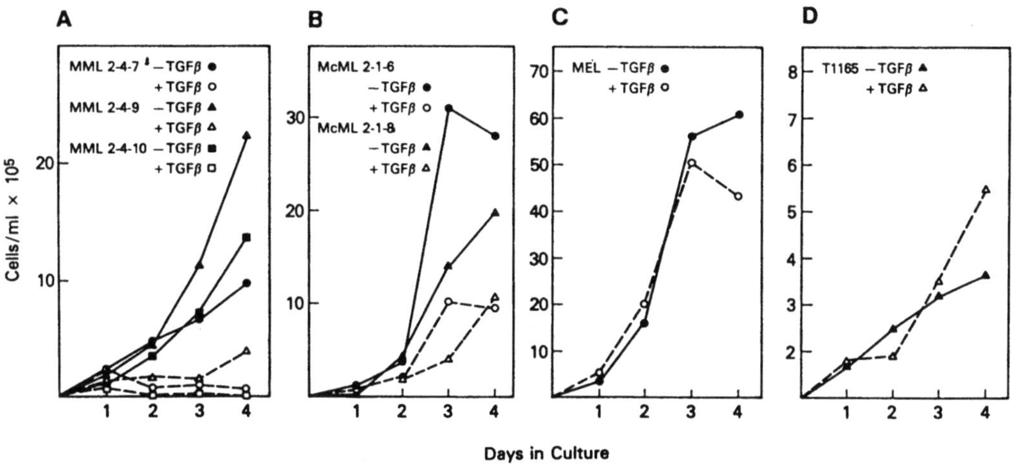

Fig. 4. Effect of TGF β on myeloid tumor cell proliferation. Cells were seeded in D-MEM supplemented with 10% FCS. In cultures containing human platelet derived TGF β1 (obtained from Joseph DeLarco (Otsuka Pharmaceutical Co., Rockville, MD),the factor was added at a concentration of 4u per ml. Panel A, promonocytic MML cells; Panel B, McML macrophage/monocyte cells; Panel C, MEL, murine erythroleukemia cells (Wolff, Tambourin, and Ruscetti 1986); Panel D, T1165, a plasmacytoma cell line, grown in the presence of P388D1 conditioned medium (Nordan and Potter 1986).

which are unaffected by TGF β were included as controls. Sensitivity to TGF β has been associated with precursor populations of myeloid cells and insensitivity has been associated with mature cells (Keller et al 1988). This difference in sensitivity as well as several other differences noted above would suggest that the MML cells are not as fully maturated along the monocytic pathway as the McML cells although they are clearly committed to the pathway. It is hoped that knowledge of these and other differences in the properties and sensitivities of the cells will eventually assist us in understanding why the two tumors respond so differently to the treatment of mice with indomethacin, a non-steroid anti-inflammatory drug. As reported recently, MML tumor induction can be inhibited 100% when the drug is added to the drinking water, whereas McML tumor induction is unaffected (Wolff et al 1988).

ACKNOWLEDGEMENT

We would like to thank Richard Koller for excellent technical assistence.

REFERENCES

Baumbach WR, Keath EJ, Cole MD (1986) A mouse c-myc retrovirus transforms established fibroblast lines in vitro and induces monocyte-macrophage tumors in vivo. J Virol 59:276-283

Gleichman E, Pals ST, Rolink AG, Radaszkiewicz T, Gleichman, H (1984) Graft-versus-host reactions (GVHR): Pathogenetic pathways to a spectrum of immunological diseases. Immunol Today 5:324-332

Reik W, Weiher H, Jaenisch R (1985) Replication-competent Moloney murine leukemia virus carrying a bacterial suppressor tRNA gene: Selective cloning of proviral and flanking host sequences. Proc Natl Acad Sci USA 82:1141-1145

Keller JR, Mantel C, Sing GK, Ellingsworth LR, Ruscetti SK, Ruscetti FW (1988) Transforming growth factor β1 selectively regulates early murine hematopoietic progenitors and inhibits the growth of IL-3 dependent myeloid leukemia cell lines. J Exp Med, In press.

Metcalf D (1984) Hemopoietic Colony Stimulating Factors. Elsevier, Amsterdam, pp 97-170

Nordan R, Potter M (1986) A macrophage-derived factor required by plasmacytomas for survival and proliferation in vitro. Science 233:566-569

Potter M (1984) Genetics of susceptibility to plasmacytoma development in BALB/c mice. Cancer Surveys 3:247-264

Potter M (1986) Plasmacytoma development in BALB/c mice. Adv Viral Oncol 7:99-12

Potter M, Mushinski, JF Mushinski EB, Brust S, Wax JS, Weiner F, Babonits M, Rapp, UR, Morse HC III (1987) Avian v-myc replaces chromosomal translocation in murine plasmacytomas. Science 235:787-789

Schwartz RS, Beldotti L (1965) Malignant lymphomas following allogeneic disease: transition from an immunological to a neoplastic disorder. Science 149:1511-1514

Shen-Ong GLC, Wolff L (1987) Moloney murine leukemia virus-induced myeloid tumors in adult BALB/c mice: Requirement of c-myb activation but lack of v-abl involvement. J Virol 61:3721-3725

Wolff L, Mushinski JF, Gilboa E, Morse HC III (1986) Induction of hematopoietic tumors using a viral construct containing c-myc cDNA from normal mouse spleen. Curr Topics Immunol 132:33-39

Wolff L, Tambourin P, Ruscetti S (1986) Induction of the autonomous stage of transformation in erythroid cells infected with SFFV: Helper virus is not required. Virol 152:272-276

Wolff L, Mushinski JF, Shen-Ong GLC, Morse HC III (1988) A chronic inflammatory response: Its role in supporting the development of c-myb and c-myc relat4d promonocytic and monocytic tumors in BALB/c mice. J Immunol 141:681-689

Studies of Secondary Transforming Events in Murine c-*myc* Retrovirus-Induced Monocyte Tumors

Michael R. Eccles, William R. Baumbach, Gregory D. Schuler, and Michael D. Cole.

Department of Molecular Biology, Princeton University, Princeton, NJ.

INTRODUCTION

Rearrangement or deregulation of the c-myc gene has been observed in a variety of tumors and transformed cell lines (reviewed by Cole, 1986). Yet, the normal function or the exact contribution of c-myc in tumorigenesis remains controversial. We have recently described a tumor system in which a c-myc retrovirus induces monocyte/macrophage tumors in pristane treated BALB/c mice with very high frequency (Baumbach et al., 1986). This system has enabled us to begin dissecting the molecular changes during c-myc induced transformation of monocytes in vivo. Expression of c-myc alone is insufficient for full tumorigenicity, and as in the case of ras cooperativity (Land et al., 1983, Ruley et al., 1983), collaboration of a second genetic activation appears to be necessary. We have shown that in at least one monocyte tumor (tumor 7.1.3), a change involving the CSF-1 gene has occurred (Baumbach et al., 1987). In this tumor an endogenous ecotropic virus has integrated just upstream of the CSF-1 gene, thus activating production of CSF-1. This tumor now grows by an autocrine mechanism. Indeed all of the tumors have aquired a degree of autonomy, and so do not require CSF-1 for growth. However, only tumor 7.1.3 can be growth inhibited by an anti CSF-1 antibody (Baumbach et al., 1987), and therefore the other tumors must be CSF-1 independent through some other mechanisms. Hence, we have continued to look for further genetic changes by which CSF-1 independence could have arisen. Here we present an update of several lines of investigation aimed at finding and understanding the role of secondary genetic changes in myc-induced monocyte tumors. We also address the question of why there is down regulation of endogenous c-myc expression following monocyte tumorigenesis.

RESULTS AND DISCUSSION.

Expression of PDGFR Related mRNA in the Monocyte Tumor 10.1.1.

The receptor for platelet-derived growth factor (PDGFR) has a strikingly similar structure to the receptor for CSF-1 (Yarden et al., 1986). Based on the initial finding that activation of the CSF-1 signal pathway can provide an important secondary genetic change in monocyte tumor progression, we hypothesized that the PDGFR gene would also be a candidate for rearrangement or activation in monocytes infected with a c-myc retrovirus. To test this hypothesis, we

Current Topics in Microbiology and Immunology, Vol. 149

hybridized a PDGFR probe (pGR102) to Northern blots prepared from poly(A) tumor and control mRNAs. As expected, a 5.3kb message (Yarden et al., 1986) was detected in fibroblast and L-cell mRNAs (Fig. 1),

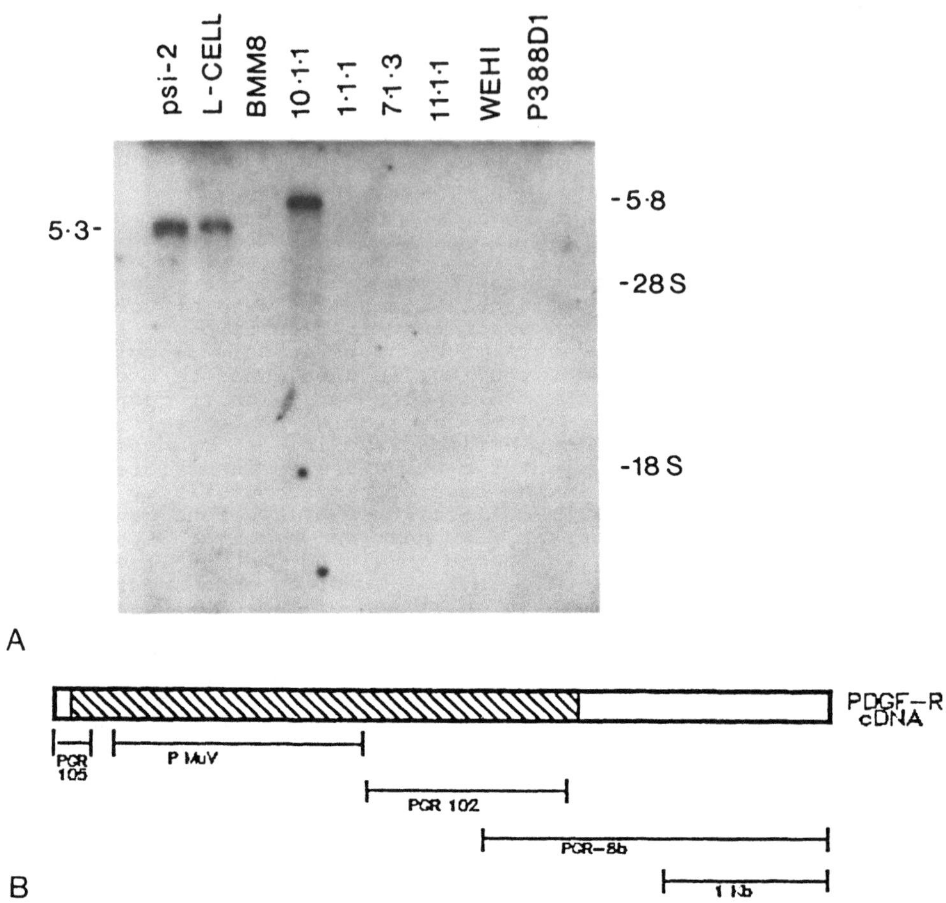

Figure 1: A) Expression of platelet-derived growth factor receptor (PDGFR) in control and tumor cell lines. Five micrograms of control and tumor poly(A) mRNA were Northern blotted and hybridized with pGR102. B) Depiction of murine fibroblast PDGFR cDNA (top) and segments which we have used to probe Northerns and Southerns containing 10.1.1 mRNA and DNA respectively. pGR105, pMuV, and pGR102 were gifts from L.T. Williams. pGR.8b is the 2.2kb cDNA which we have isolated from 10.1.1 tumor cells.

but a hybridizing band was also detected at approximately 5.8kb in tumor 10.1.1 mRNA. No other tumor lines or myc-immortalized monocytes (BMM8) expressed the PDGFR gene, indicating that this gene is not normally expressed in this cell lineage. The increased size of the mRNA in tumor 10.1.1 suggests that there may be a structural alteration of PDGFR or altered splicing of the message. To determine whether other regions of the murine PDGFR gene also hybridize to the 10.1.1 transcript, we hybridized with probes as depicted in Fig 1b. All probes hybridized to the same 5.8 kb transcript in 10.1.1, and did not reveal DNA rearrangements in a Southern blot with 10.1.1 DNA (data not shown). This suggests that the entire PDGFR coding region may be represented in the abnormal PDGFR mRNA expressed in 10.1.1.

To elucidate why the tumor-specific PDGFR transcript is larger than in fibroblasts, we have begun to isolate cDNA clones. A library of $1.2x10^6$ recombinant oligo dT primed cDNAs cloned in kGT10 were screened using pGR102 as a probe. Two clones were plaque purified, one of which yielded a 2.2kb cDNA. Comparison of the restriction map with the published sequence (Yarden et al., 1986) confirmed the identity of this clone as murine PDGFR and indicated that there has probably been no structural rearrangement in the region of the gene encoding the isolated cDNA, which covers approximately one-half of the mRNA and extends to the polyadenylation signal. We are currently pursuing further cDNA cloning to isolate the remaining sequences. Expression of PDGFR in 10.1.1 is clearly of interest with regard to receptor biology and gene regulation because PDGFR is not detectably expressed in monocytes or in cells of the same lineage at an earlier stage such as in WEHI 3B. Macrophages are, however, known to express two forms of platelet-derived growth factor (PDGF), one of which is related to the PDGF B-chain (Shimokado et al., 1985). Whether the combined expression of PDGF and a form of its receptor in 10.1.1 could result in autocrine growth stimulation is a matter to be resolved. Recent evidence suggests that, in humans at least, homodimers of the PDGF B-chain may interact with two receptors; one of which binds all three dimeric molecules, and a different receptor which binds B-B homodimers alone (Hart et al., 1988). The receptor which has been cloned from mouse and human fibroblasts may be the form which can bind all three types of PDGF (Escobedo et al., 1988). It will be of interest to determine which forms of PDGF interact with the receptor activated in tumor 10.1.1.

Re-creation of the secondary events in vitro.

One aim of our research is to determine the nature and number of events which are required to transform monocytes to malignancy. Our preliminary results suggest that, in the simplest model, no more than two genetic events need to occur. The first event in our system (integration of the c-*myc* retrovirus) is always constant and can be introduced into cells both *in vitro* or *in vivo*. The second event, which we presume leads to clonality of the tumors, occurs spontaneously during the 8 to 10 week incubation period *in vivo*. Since we have identified one, and possibly two, secondary events that appear to provide the necessary deregulation in growth control to induce the formation of monocyte/macrophage tumors *in vivo*, the question arises; can we re-create the same or similar events in vitro, and thus confirm our hypothesis by transforming monocytes to a fully tumorigenic state with two genetically engineered events. To address this question, we have isolated monocytes partially transformed by the c-myc retrovirus from two different sources: 1) Bone marrow cells cultured in vitro in CSF-1 (BMM8); 2) Peritoneal macrophages cultured in vitro in CSF-1 (PMM8). All of these cells were still dependent on exogenous CSF-1 for growth in culture. Cells were also established in culture (PMT, 7.1.3, 9.1.1) from mice with clear evidence of neoplasia (swollen abdomen, lethargy). The latter cells could grow immediately after isolation in the absence of exogenous CSF-1. To produce autonomous cells with a second genetic change in vitro, BMM8 cells were super-infected with viruses containing constitutively expressed v-fms (BMFM), GM-CSF (BMGM), or v-H-ras (BMM8ras) genes. The malignant potential of each of these cells or the c-myc only parental cells was then assessed by injection into pristane or non-pristane treated syngeneic BALB/c recipients. All retroviral infections employed helper-free virus stocks to prevent cross-infection of resident cells.

Table 1: Tumorigenicity of monocyte cell lines and tumors in pristane or non-pristane treated mice.

Cell line	Number of mice	No. of cells injected[a]	Average tumor latency (days)[b] with pristane	without pristane
BMM8	10	5×10^6	36.7	>200
BMM8	5	5×10^5	60.2	>200
BMM8	10	2.5×10^4	72.0	>200
BMFM	10	$5x10^6/1x10^6$	30.6	103 (6 mice)[c]
BMGM	10	$5x10^6/1x10^6$	31.0	108 (7 mice)
BMM8ras	10	2×10^6	N.D.	38.8 (4 mice)
PMM8	5	1×10^6	58.0	153.8
PM6A	10	1×10^6	41.5	80.9
PMT	9	1×10^6	27.8	34.0 (6 mice)
7.1.3	5	5×10^6	25.0	N.D.
9.1.1	5	5×10^6	26.4	N.D.

[a] The indicated number of cells suspended in 1.0 ml of phosphate buffered saline were injected intraperitoneally. Mice were either pretreated with 0.5 to 1.0 ml pristane i.p. 7-14 days earlier, or not pretreated at all.
[b] Tumor latency represents the time required for the tumor cells to kill the mouse.
[c] The number of mice indicated in brackets is the number of mice that died within the observation period (>200 days).

The results (Table 1) demonstrate distinct differences in the malignant potential of each cell type. The tumor cells (PMT, 7.1.3, 9.1.1) were rapidly tumorigenic and formed lethal ascites tumors in non-pristane animals (average latency 3-5 wks), whereas cells without a second event (PMM8, BMM8) are much reduced in this capacity (either non-tumorigenic or inducing tumors with an average latency of 22 wks). All of the cells were tumorigenic in pristane-treated animals. Super-infection of c-myc-immortalized monocytes with v-fms, GM-CFS, or v-H-ras containing viruses rendered these cells more malignant, i.e. they were tumorigenic in non-pristane mice, although with a longer

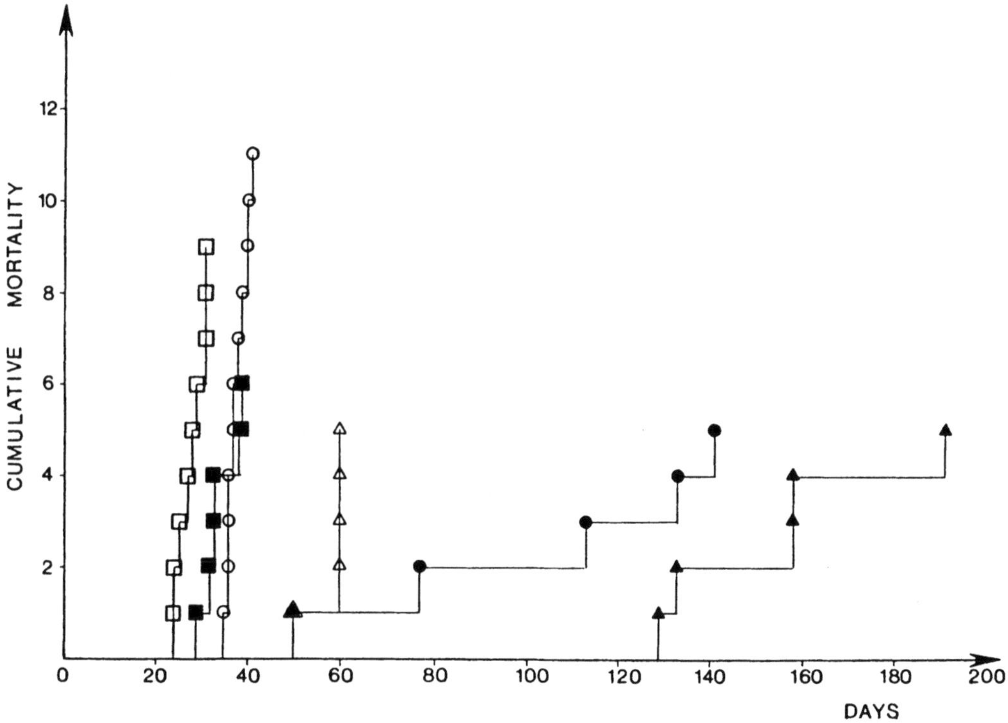

Figure 2: Cumulative mortality curves of pristane and non-pristane treated mice injected with MRV-infected macrophages. Pristane (open symbols) or non-pristane treated (closed symbols) BALB/c mice were injected with 10^6 cells into the peritoneum; PMM8 (triangles), PMT (squares), or PM6A (circles). PMM8 cells are in vitro infected, immortalized, peritoneal macrophages. PMT and PM6A cells are derived from the peritoneal washes of pristane treated BALB/c mice infected intraperitoneally with a myc retrovirus, and which have a tumor (PMT) or do not have a tumor (PM6A) at six weeks post-infection. PMT and PM6A are immortalized, but are CSF-1 independent and dependent respectively.

latency (~100d) than tumor cells which arise in vivo (~35d). The simplest interpretation of these results is that the expression of a c-myc oncogene and a cooperating second gene induces a malignant state similar to, but possibly distinct from, that arising in vivo.

It should be noted that the CSF-1-dependent BMM8 cells are tumorigenic in pristane-treated mice, but not in the absence of pristane. We interpret this result to indicate that the large number of partially transformed cells innoculated into a "permissive" environment allows the rapid outgrowth of malignant cells. In every case, the tumor cells arising from BMM8 cells had become CSF-1-independent for growth in culture, apparently mimicing the tumors that arise from direct virus infection. The BMM8 cells cannot form tumors in the absence of the microenvironment induced by pristane treatment.

We wished to explore this simplistic two event model further and to test for more subtle differences in the transformed phenotype of pre-malignant cells arising in vivo. To this end, two pristane-treated mice were injected with MRV and peritoneal cells (PM6A) were obtained at 6 weeks post infection. These cells were partially transformed in that they could be cultured indefinitely in vitro, but the cells were still dependent on CSF-1 (data not shown). PM6A cells were cultured for 4 weeks and then re-injected into pristane-treated or non-pristane mice. For comparison, additional mice were injected with PMM8 or PMT cells. The cumulative motality curves, shown in Fig. 2, suggest that peritoneal MRV infected monocytes isolated at 6 weeks post infection (PM6A) are more tumorigenic than their in vitro c-myc retrovirus-infected counterparts (PMM8 or BMM8). Both cell lines are, however, much less tumorigenic in non-pristane treated mice. These results suggest a more complicated scenario than the two-event model discussed above. Apparently, CSF-1-dependent cells arise in vivo that are more malignant than those generated in vitro. On the other hand, it should be noted that the latency with which PM6A causes tumors in pristane-treated mice is equivalent to that resulting from a 10-fold increase in the number of BMM8 cells injected. This data may indicate that some relatively common changes are occurring during in vivo tumor progression that can predispose the cells to secondary genetic changes. Defining, in molecular terms, the nature of this progression may allow a better understanding of in vivo myeloid tumorigenesis.

Expression of the endogenous myc gene in myc-induced macrophage tumors.

Down-regulation of the endogenous c-myc gene has been observed in many tumors induced by the c-myc oncogene, including the monocyte tumors described in this study (Baumbach et al., 1987). The mechanism by which c-myc is down regulated in tumor cells remains uncertain and several models have been proposed to account for this phenomenon. One model proposes that the high level of c-myc protein from the activated gene feeds back in an auto-regulatory loop and shuts off transcription from the proto-oncogene (Leder et al., 1983). However, many studies indicate that cells which have been transfected with viral promoter linked c-myc genes show normal levels of endogenous c-myc mRNA levels

(Keath et al., 1984; Coppola and Cole, 1986). A second proposal is that the activated c-myc gene has more stable mRNA than the normal c-myc mRNA, which is degraded very rapidly (Piechacazyk et al., 1985; Rabbitts et al., 1985). A third suggestion is that down regulation of c-myc expression is linked to the developmental stage of the cells in which the tumors arise.

Myc-induced macrophage tumors provide an ideal system to explore whether the c-myc proto-oncogene is down-regulated due to transcriptional or post-transcriptional processes because the first exon of c-myc is not contained within the c-myc virus, unlike plasmacytomas or Burkitts lymphomas where the translocated first exon can complicate the interpretation of the data. Run-on transcription was used to determine whether the monocyte tumors transcribe the endogenous myc proto-oncogene. Two separate subcloned regions of the mouse c-myc gene were used as probes, i.e. equivalent sized fragments from the first and second exons of c-myc. The integrated provirus only contains exons 2 and 3 so the signal from the exon 1 probe represents expression of the endogenous gene. Other genes hybridized as probes were fos, KC, histone H3 (as a positive control) and pBR322 (negative control). The results show that hybridization to the first exon probe is much reduced in the monocyte tumors (Fig. 3). This implies that down-regulation of c-myc in myc-induced monocyte tumors is due to decreased transcription. Somewhat unexpectedly, there was a lower level of hybridization to the exon 2 probe in the tumors than in the P388D1 cell line, even though the level of cytoplasmic mRNA from

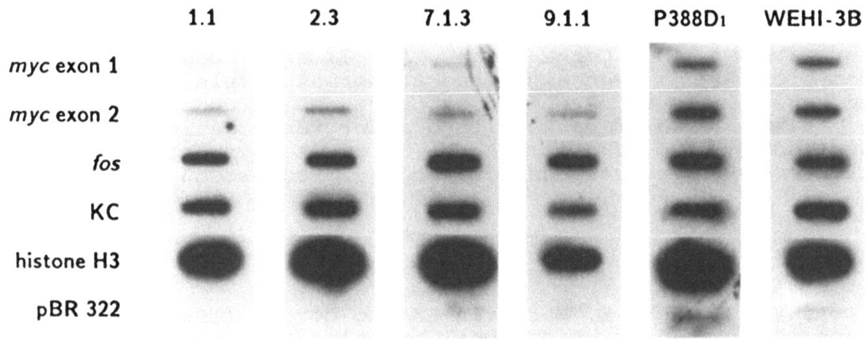

Figure 3: The endogenous c-myc gene is not transcribed in macrophage tumors. Run-on transcription assays were performed on macrophage tumors 1.1, 2.3, 7.1.3, and 9.1.1. The radiolabelled transcription products were then hybridized to filters containing c-myc first exon (subcloned 0.46 kb BamH1-Bgl II fragment), c-myc second exon (subcloned 0.58 kb Pst 1 fragment), fos (1.3 kb region of FBJ MuLV homologous to c-fos), KC (full-length cDNA - 0.5 kb), histone H3 (a complete mouse gene - 0.54 kb), and the plasmid pBR322 (as a negative control).

the proviral c-myc gene is quite high (Baumbach et al., 1987). This is probably due to an overall lower level of transcription from the proviral gene, but a much longer half-lives of the proviral transcripts (>4 hours compared with normal c-myc mRNA which decays with a half-life of <30 minutes; unpublished results). The proviral mRNA lacks the 3' untranslated region that has been shown to contribute to instability of c-myc mRNA (Jones and Cole, 1987). Further experiments have demonstrated that the c-myc proto-oncogene in the myc-induced tumors is not inducible by a wide variety of bio-active compounds including TPA, Bt_2-cAMP, or cyclohexamide (G. Schuler, submitted). The inability to reactivate the silent endogenous c-myc gene may indicate that the gene is irreversibly down-regulated upon differentiation. Thus we favor the third model mentioned above, i.e. that the tumors arise at a stage in development during which the normal c-myc gene is inactive.

From the results we have presented above, it is apparent that murine BALB/c macrophages infected with our c-myc retrovirus are pre-tumorigenic, and require a second cooperating genetic alteration to become tumorigenic in non-pristane mice. Our experiments have largely shown that deregulated growth factor or growth factor receptor genes can provide this additional event, allowing an alternative mechanism for cell growth other than the normal CSF-1 responsive pathway. However, using in vitro studies with mice infected six weeks prior to recovery of myc-infected peritoneal cells, we have preliminary evidence that a two genetic event model may be an oversimplification. If this is true, what are the additional events? It would seem that progression to malignancy can be quite rapid, and that the rate limiting steps of tumorigenesis appear to be largely overcome with the introduction of a c-myc oncogene and a deregulated growth factor pathway gene. Cerni et al., (1987) have suggested that a deregulated myc oncogene, even expressed at normal levels, may induce an increased rate of sister chromatid exchange and chromosomal alterations. Thus, clones of cells with greater tumorigenicity may be quickly generated in vivo, and it will be of great interest to identify which changes are responsible for the progression to malignancy.

REFERENCES

Adams J, Gerondakis S, Webb E, Corcoran LM and Cory S (1983) Cellular myc oncogene is altered by chromosomal translocation to the immunuglobulin locus in murine plasmacytomas and is rearranged similarly in human Burkitt lymphomas. Proc. Natl. Acad. Sci. USA 80: 1982-1986

Baumbach WR, Keath EJ, Cole MD (1986) A mouse c-myc retrovirus transforms established fibroblast lines in vitro and induces monocyte/macrophage tumors in vivo. J. Virol. 59: 276-283

Baumbach WR, Stanley ER, Cole MD (1987) Induction of clonal monocyte-macrophage tumors in vivo by a mouse c-myc retrovirus: Rearrangement of the CSF-1 gene as a secondary transforming event. Mol. Cell. Biol. 7: 664-671

Cerni C, Mogneau E, Cuzins F (1987) Transfer of "immortalizing" oncogenes into rat fibroblasts induces both high rates of sister chromatid exchange and appearance of abnormal karyotypes. Exp. Cell Res. 168: 439-446

Cole MD (1986) The myc oncogene: its role in transformation and differentiation. Annu. Rev. Genet. 20: 361-384

Coppola JA and Cole MD (1986) Constitutive c-myc expression blocks murine erythroleukemia cell differentiation but not commitment. Nature 320: 760-763

Escobedo JA, Navankasatussas S, Coussens LS, Coughlin SR, Bell GI, Williams LT (1988) A common PDGF receptor is activated by homodimeric A and B forms of PDGF. Science 240: 1532-1534

Hart CE, Forstram JW, Kelly JD, Seifert RA, Smith RA, Ross R, Murray MJ, Bowen-Pope DF (1988) Two classes of PDGF receptor recognize different isoforms of PDGF. Science 240: 1529-1531

Jones TR, and Cole MD (1987) Rapid cytoplasmic turnover of c-myc mRNA: Requirement of the 3' untranslated sequences. Mol. Cell. Biol. 7: 4513-4521

Keath EJ, Caimi PG, Cole MD (1984) Fibroblast lines expressing activated c-myc oncogenes are tumorigenic in nude mice and syngeneic animals. Cell 39: 339-348

Land H, Parada LF, Weinberg RA (1983) Tumorigenic conversion of primary embryo fibroblasts requires at least two cooperating oncogenes. Nature 304: 596-602

Leder P, Battey J, Lenoir G, Moulding C, Murphy W, Potter H, Stewart T, Taub R (1983) Translocations among antibody genes in human cancer. Science 222: 765-771

Piechaczyk M, Yang YQ, Blanchard JM, Jeanteur P, Marcu KB (1985) Posttranscriptional mechanisms are responsible for accumulation of truncated c-myc RNAs in murine plasmacytoma cells. Cell 42: 589-597

Rabbits PH, Forester A, Stinson MA, Rabbits TH (1985) Truncation of exon 1 from the c-myc gene results in prolonged c-myc mRNA stability. EMBO J. 4: 3727-3733

Ruley HE (1983) Adenovirus early region 1A enables viral cellular transforming genes to transform primary cells in culture. Nature 304: 602-606

Shimokado K, Raines EW, Madtes DK, Barret TB, Benditt EP, Ross R (1985) A significant part of macrophage-derived growth factor consists of at least two forms of PDGF. Cell 43: 277-286

Stanton LW, Watt R, Marcu KB (1983) Nucleotide sequence composition of normal and translocated murine c-myc genes. Nature 310: 423-425

Yarden Y, Escobedo JA, Kuang W-J, Yang-Feng TL, Daniel TO, Tremble PM, Chen EY, Ando ME, Harkins RN, Francke U, Fried VA, Ullrich A, Williams LT (1986) Structure of the receptor for platelet-derived growth factor helps define a family of closely related growth factor receptors. Nature 323: 226-231

Analysis of the Leukemogenic Properties of the *bcr*-v-*abl* and GM-CSF Genes Using a New Retroviral Vector

I. K. Hariharan, G. R. Johnson, T. J. Gonda*, D. Metcalf, J. M. Adams and S. Cory

The Walter and Eliza Hall Institute of Medical Research and *Ludwig Institute of Cancer Research, Melbourne Tumour Biology Branch, P. O. Royal Melbourne Hospital 3050, Melbourne, Australia

INTRODUCTION

The haemopoietic system consists of a hierarchy of cells that are produced throughout life from a small number of self renewing stem cells. Many of the molecules that regulate normal haemopoiesis have been defined and characterized by studying aspects of haemopoiesis that can occur in vitro under controlled conditions. Furthermore, our knowledge of the haemopoietic system has been supplemented by investigations of disease phenomena where haemopoiesis is perturbed. These include naturally occurring leukaemias in humans and those induced experimentally in laboratory animals.

We have investigated the effects of the expression of an oncogene and the aberrant expression of a growth factor gene on haemopoietic cells. To that end we first developed a new retroviral vector that was capable of expressing the introduced genes at high levels both in vitro and in vivo.

A NEW RETROVIRAL VECTOR

To facilitate efficient expression in haemopoietic cells, we used a new retroviral vector, pMPZen (Hariharan, Adams and Cory, submitted) which was derived from the previously described vector pMPZipNeo (Bowtell et al., 1987) as outlined in Figure 1. Both vectors utilize the enhancer sequence from the myeloproliferative sarcoma virus (MPSV), which allows elevated expression within myeloid cells (Bowtell et al., 1988). With the pMPZen vector, the introduced gene is expressed from the spliced (subgenomic) mRNA, as is the Neo gene in the Zip-based vectors and the env gene in natural murine leukaemia viruses. This design was prompted by our observation that Zip-based viruses bearing only the Neo gene were transcribed well in cultured haemopoietic cell lines and in mice repopulated from infected multipotential stem cells, whereas derivatives carrying an additional gene within the 5' (BamHI) cloning site were expressed very poorly (Bowtell et al., 1987; 1988). The spliced RNA lacks several ATG codons that lie upstream of the BamHI site and which may impede translation. In some experiments we used a version of pMPZen that carries within its 3' region the Neo selectable marker driven by the SV40 enhancer/early promoter - pMPZenSVNeo (Figure 1). Cells infected with this virus can be selected in G418-containing media, independently of any properties of the inserted gene.

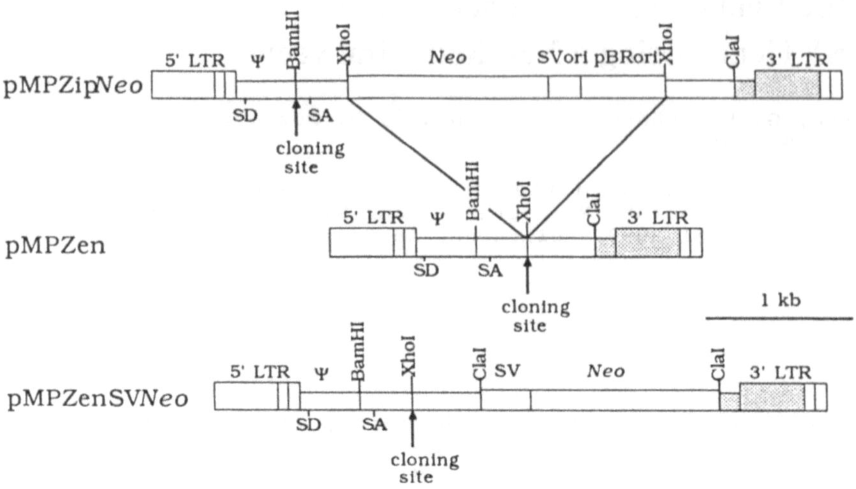

Figure 1 Construction of pMPZen and pMPZenSVNeo
SD and SA denote splice donor and splice acceptor respectively. The stippled region was derived from MPSV.

CONSTITUTIVE PRODUCTION OF GM-CSF IN VIVO PRODUCES A FATAL MYELOPROLIFERATIVE SYNDROME

A class of genes that are likely to participate in leukaemogenesis are those that code for the colony stimulating factors (CSF). As most myeloid cells express receptors for some of these regulators, it is conceivable that a leukaemia can arise when a myeloid cell begins to secrete CSF. Indeed, cells of the factor-dependent myeloid cell line FDC-P1 can be rendered factor independent and leukaemogenic when they produce their own granulocyte-macrophage colony stimulating factor (GM-CSF)(Lang et al., 1985).

GM-CSF Expression Facilitates Autonomous Proliferation

To study the effects of GM-CSF expression in normal haemopoietic cells, the GM-CSF cDNA was inserted into the MPZen retroviral vector. A significant portion of the 3′ untranslated region, which includes a sequence that accelerates degradation of mRNA (Shaw and Kamen, 1986), was removed from the cDNA clone (Gough et al., 1987). Helper-free virus producing lines were generated by transfecting the retroviral plasmid into the ψ-2 packaging line (Mann et al., 1983).

When foetal liver cells were co-cultivated with cells producing the MPZen(GM-CSF) virus and subsequently plated in medium lacking an exogenous source of CSF, cell proliferation was evident for up to 18 weeks. In contrast, cells in mock-infected control cultures died within 10 days. Most of the proliferating cells resembled macrophages and secreted GM-CSF into the growth medium. Despite their apparent autonomy *in vitro*, these cells failed to form tumours in syngeneic mice.

Foetal liver or bone marrow cells infected with the MPZen(GM-CSF) virus generated colonies which grew in agar in the absence of an exogenous source of CSF. The composition of colonies on day 7 was identical to those generated from normal progenitors stimulated by GM-CSF (neutrophils and/or macrophages with occasional eosinophils). Some of the colonies continued to proliferate when transferred into liquid culture and generated long-lived GM-CSF-secreting macrophages.

In order to infect multipotential haemopoietic cells, marrow from mice injected with 5-fluorouracil was co-cultivated with the virus-producing ψ-2 cells and injected into lethally-irradiated recipients. Almost all (9 of 10) colonies dissected from spleens of mice sacrificed 12-14 days after receiving marrow harboured the provirus. These spleen colonies contained variable proportions of erythroid, granulocyte, macrophage, megakaryocyte, eosinophil and blast cells, indicating that they derived from multipotential cells. Infected spleen colonies secreted GM-CSF and some generated factor-independent colonies in agar, indicating that they contained factor-independent progenitor cells.

GM-CSF Expression Perturbs Haemopoiesis *in vivo*.

To determine if production of GM-CSF by haemopoietic cells perturbs their differentiation *in vivo*, lethally-irradiated mice were transplanted with 10^6 post-5-FU bone marrow cells which had been co-cultivated with the MPZen(GM-CSF) virus-producing line. While control mice repopulated with bone marrow co-cultivated with ψ-2 cells remained healthy for 6 months, all mice receiving the GM-CSF virus-infected cells became severely ill 2 to 3 weeks after transplantation and none survived after 4 weeks.

Detailed examination of the virus-bearing mice confirmed that the disease was a consequence of excessive production of GM-CSF. Very high levels of GM-CSF activity were detected in the sera of virus-infected animals and medium conditioned by their bone marrow, spleen and peritoneal cells. Southern and Northern blot analysis revealed that these cells harboured the provirus (on average, 1-2 copies per cell) and expressed the viral RNAs (2.5 and 2.0 kb). The mice contained strikingly increased numbers of neutrophils, monocytes, macrophages and eosinophils in the bone marrow, spleen, peripheral blood and peritoneal cavity. Surprisingly, the number of progenitor cells (GM-CFC) in bone marrow was reduced when compared to the controls although up to 76% of the GM-CFC were factor independent.

Histological examination revealed extensive invasion of many organs by mitotically-active granulocytes and macrophages, most notably the lungs and the liver. The accumulations in the lungs were focal and often replaced all the tissue in a lobe. Periportal and diffuse infiltration was evident in the liver (Figure 2) and infiltration and tissue destruction were evident in the heart, skeletal muscle, retina and sometimes the femur. Remarkably, the thymus was invariably devoid of lymphoid cells in the cortex and contained only small numbers of lymphoid cells in the medulla, in marked contrast to the essentially normal thymus seen in control mice. Several lymph nodes were depleted of lymphoid cells and instead were infiltrated by granulocytes or macrophages. While these observations raise the intriguing possibility that GM-CSF expression can alter the lineage commitment of multipotential cells to favour myelopoiesis rather than lymphopoiesis, this phenomenon may merely reflect an inhibitory effect on lymphopoiesis by the massive myeloproliferation.

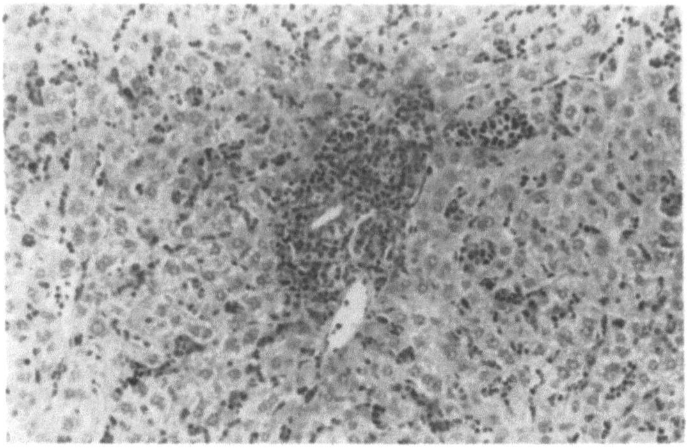

Figure 2 Infiltration of the liver with granulocytes and macrophages.

The myeloproliferative disease was not transplantable. Bone marrow, spleen or peritoneal cells from primary recipients failed to produce tumours when transplanted into sub-lethally irradiated or unirradiated secondary recipients even up to 44 weeks after transplantation. Furthermore, none of the recipients had elevated numbers of white cells in their peripheral blood or elevated levels of GM-CSF in their urine.

Expression of GM-CSF in haemopoietic cells can thus result in a fatal myeloproliferative syndrome. As cells from various stages of differentiation were likely to have been infected and transplanted together with uninfected cells, the pathological changes probably reflect changes in each of these populations. Altered lineage commitment of multipotential cells, an incresed rate of proliferation of committed progenitors and an increased life span of mature cells could all contribute to the observed phenotype. The high serum level of GM-CSF achieved is likely to enhance the proliferation and/or survival of non-infected cells of the granulocyte-macrophage lineages. This polyclonal myeloproliferation is reminiscent of several human haemopoietic disorders that predispose to myeloid leukaemia including juvenile chronic myeloid leukaemia and refractory anaemia with excess blasts. Introduction of other growth factor genes or known oncogenes into these mice may mimic the evolution of a frank leukaemia.

bcr-v-abl AND MYELOID LEUKAEMIA: A POTENTIAL AUTOCRINE MECHANISM

Much progress has been made over the last five years in the molecular definition of the genetic lesion that occurs in patients with chronic myeloid leukaemia (CML). The leukaemic cells contain an activated allele of the c-abl oncogene which has been generated by the fusion of sequences coded by the 5′ portion of the bcr gene to the 3′ exons of abl to form a hybrid bcr-abl gene (Shtivelman et al., 1985; Grosveld et al., 1986). The resulting bcr-abl polypeptide resembles the onco-protein of the Abelson murine leukaemia virus in that it has enhanced autophosphorylation activity *in vitro* and is phosphorylated on tyrosine *in vivo* (Konopka et al., 1984). Formation of the hybrid gene is hence likely to represent a crucial event in the pathogenesis of CML.

We constructed a synthetic bcr-v-abl which mimics the bcr-c-abl gene found in CML by fusing bcr sequences coding for the N-terminal 827 amino acid residues (Hariharan and Adams, 1987) to v-abl sequences from the p120 form of the Abelson virus (Hariharan et al., submitted). The bcr-v-abl gene was cloned into the XhoI site of the pMPZenSVNeo vector. In order to make a helper-free bcr-v-abl virus, the bcr-v-abl retroviral construct was transfected into ψ2 fibroblasts. This experiment also permitted us to assess the effects of bcr-v-abl expression upon fibroblast cells. Two clones expressing bcr-v-abl retained the relatively flat non-transformed morphology of the parental ψ2 cells. In contrast, ψ2 cells that harbour an Abelson provirus and express a gag-v-abl protein are round and refractile and grow in a semi-adherent manner. When ψ-abl cells were injected into nude mice they produced large tumours at the site of injection within 14 days. In contrast, neither of the ψ-bcr-v-abl clones had produced tumours even after three months. Thus, like the bcr-c-abl gene, (Daley et al., 1987), the bcr-v-abl construct does not transform fibroblasts.

bcr-v-abl renders FDC-P1 cells factor independent

In order to examine the effects of the altered abl genes upon haemopoietic cells, we infected a clonal derivative of the myeloid cell line FDC-P1 (Dexter et al., 1980) with either AMuLV or the bcr-v-abl virus. FDC-P1 is an immature murine myeloid cell line that requires either IL-3 (Multi-CSF) or GM-CSF for growth in culture. It has been shown previously that infection with AMuLV abrogates the factor requirement of FDC-P1 cells and renders them tumourigenic in syngeneic mice (Cook et al., 1985). FDC-P1 cells were cocultivated with virus-producing ψ2 cells, washed and plated either in agar or in liquid culture in both the presence and absence of WEHI3B conditioned medium (W3CM) - a source of IL-3.

Factor-independent cells were obtained from cultures of FDC-P1 cells exposed to either AMuLV or the bcr-v-abl virus but not from control cultures of mock-infected FDC-P1 cells (Table 1). To establish whether cells selected solely by their G418-resistance were also factor independent, six G418-resistant clones were expanded in liquid medium containing IL-3, and then replated in soft agar with and without W3CM. For all six clones, the absence of exogenous IL-3 made no difference to the colony frequency, suggesting that most, if not all, G418-resistant cells are factor independent. Furthermore, all factor-independent clones analysed harboured an intact provirus and expressed the appropriate RNA species. Hence the factor-independent phenotype is generated by expression of the bcr-v-abl gene and does not require some rare genetic alteration.

Table I. Infection of FDC-P1 Cells: Incidence of G418-Resistant and Factor-Independent Colonies.

Viral gene	Selection W3CM	Selection G418	Colonies/10^5 cells
bcr-v-abl	+	−	16,300
	−	−	150
	+	+	31
	−	+	25
gag-v-abl	+	−	15,300
	−	−	583
	+	+	0
	−	+	0
Nil[a]	+	−	10,000
	−	−	0
	+	+	0
	−	+	0

[a] FDC-P1 cells co-cultivated with parental ψ-2 cells.

When 10^6 cells from four bcr-v-abl virus-infected clones were injected into syngeneic (DBA/2) mice, each of the cell lines produced tumours, usually within 21 days of injection, as did 10^6 cells from factor-independent clones generated with AMuLV. In contrast, mice injected with 10^7 parental FDC-P1 cells had not developed tumours even six months after injection.

Factor-independent Cells Grow in a Density-independent Manner but Make Trace Amounts of a Growth Factor

Is the factor-independent growth due to autocrine production of a growth factor? Growth was not retarded at low cell density, as the plating efficiency of two factor-independent cell lines was unaffected by the initial cell density or by inclusion of growth factor in the medium. Furthermore single cells micromanipulated into 0.25 ml cultures were capable of proliferation. Thus fully autonomous proliferation occurs even at extremely low cell density.

When poly-A^+ RNA from factor-independent cells was analysed by Northern blot hybridization, neither IL-3 nor GM-CSF mRNA was detected. However, when media conditioned by the factor-independent lines were concentrated 30X by ultrafiltration and assayed in microcultures, all the lines released an activity that could sustain the proliferation of 32Dcl.23 cells. The factor production must have resulted from the infection, because medium conditioned by the parental FDC-P1 cells (grown in recombinant GM-CSF) was unable to sustain the proliferation of 32Dcl.23 cells even after a 25-fold concentration (Duhrsen, 1988). Hence both bcr-v-abl and the Abelson oncogene appear to have induced production of low levels of a myeloid growth factor.

The induced factor is almost certainly IL-3 as that is the only factor known to permit 32Dcl.23 cells to proliferate (Hapel et al., 1981). Moreover, we found that an antiserum directed against IL-3 completely inhibited the ability of conditioned media from two factor-independent cell lines to stimulate the proliferation of FDC-P1 cells. To monitor any non-specific cytotoxicity of antibody for the target cells, control FDC-P1 cultures growing in the presence of GM-CSF as the stimulus were also tested. No non-specific inhibition was observed.

In order to ascertain whether an antiserum directed against IL-3 could inhibit the proliferation of the factor-independent cell lines, approximately 30 cells from a line infected with AMuLV and two lines expressing bcr-v-abl were cultured in microwells with an anti-IL-3 serum at a concentration that completely inhibited the IL-3-dependent proliferation of FDC-P1 cells. The antiserum had no effect on the growth of any of the factor-independent lines.

Mechanism of Factor Independence

The factor-independent cells derived by infection with the bcr-v-abl or Abelson virus grow in a density-independent manner and their growth at high dilution is unaltered by the addition of exogenous factor indicating that their proliferation is already maximally stimulated. The classic autocrine model cannot account for these properties. While it is possible that viral infection elicited a constitutive proliferative signal independent of growth factor, it seems significant that all the transformed clones make small amounts of a factor that can stimulate proliferation of the parental cells. Since the rate of diffusion of the secreted factor is likely to be low, its concentration at the surface of the cell may well be high enough to stimulate proliferation maximally. Alternatively, the factor may interact with the receptor within an intracellular compartment, as suggested previously for GM-CSF (Lang et al., 1985). In any case, the signal elicited by small amounts of bound factor may well be amplified by abl-induced alterations to the transduction pathway.

Is the mechanism of transformation of FDC-P1 cells by bcr-v-abl similar to that which occurs in CML? Progenitor cells from patients with CML have an absolute requirement for an exogenous CSF for proliferation *in vitro* (see Metcalf, 1985). The primary lesion in CML, however, *probably* occurs in a self-renewing stem cell, which in this property at least resembles some of the immortal cell lines such as FDC-P1. Due to the immense clonal expansion inherent in normal haemopoietic differentiation, even a minor growth advantage to a stem cell would lead to the emergence of a dominant clone. Hence the autocrine production of even minute amounts of a stem cell growth factor might well be sufficient to maintain the cell in a cycling state and thus engender the leukaemic clone. In order to dissect the role of the bcr-abl gene in the pathogenesis of CML *in* vivo, we are currently repopulating mice with bone marrow infected with a high-titre MPZen virus expressing the hybrid gene.

REFERENCES

Bowtell DDL, Johnson GR, Kelso A, Cory S (1987) Expression of genes transferred to haemopoietic stem cells by recombinant retroviruses. Mol Biol Med 4:229-250

Bowtell DDL, Cory S, Johnson GR, Gonda TJ (1988) A comparison of expression in hemopoietic cells by retroviral vectors carrying two genes. J Virol 62:2464-2473

Cook WD, Metcalf D, Nicola NA, Burgess AW, Walker F (1985) Malignant transformation of a growth factor-dependent myeloid cell line by Abelson virus without evidence of an autocrine mechanism. Cell 41:677-683.

Daley GQ, McLaughlin J, Witte ON, Baltimore D (1987) The CML-specific P210 bcr/abl protein, unlike v-abl does not transform NIH/3T3 fibroblasts. Science 237:532-535

Dexter TM, Garland J, Scott D, Scolnick E, Metcalf D (1980) Growth of factor-dependent hemopoietic precursor cell lines. J Exp Med 152:1036-1047.

Duhrsen U (1988) In vitro growth patterns and autocrine production of hemopoietic colony stimulating factors: analysis of leukemic populations arising in irradiated mice from cells of an injected factor-dependent continuous cell line. Leukemia 2:334-342

Gough NM, Grail D, Gearing DP, Metcalf D (1987) Mutagenesis of murine granulocyte-macrophage colony stimulating factor reveals critical residues near the N-terminus. Eur J Biochem 169:353-358

Grosveld G, Verwoerd T, Van Agthoven T, De Klein A, Ramachandran KL, Heisterkamp N, Stam K, Groffen J (1986) The chronic myelocytic cell line K562 contains a breakpoint in bcr and produces a chimeric bcr/c-abl transcript. Mol Cell Biol 6:607-616

Hapel AJ, Lee JC, Farrar WL, Ihle JN (1981) Different colony stimulating factors are detected by the IL-3 dependent cell lines FDC-P1 and 32Dcl-23. Blood 46:786-790.

Hariharan IK, Adams JM (1987) cDNA sequence for human bcr, the gene that translocates to the abl oncogene in chronic myeloid leukaemia EMBO J 6:115-119

Hariharan IK, Adams JM, Cory S bcr-v-abl oncogene renders myeloid cell line factor independent: potential autocrine mechanism in chronic myeloid leukaemia. (submitted)

Konopka JB, Watanabe SM, Witte ON (1984) An alteration of the human c-abl protein in K562 leukemia cells unmasks associated tyrosine kinase activity. Cell 37:1035-1042

Lang RA, Matcalf D, Gough NM, Dunn AR, Gonda TJ (1985) Expression of a hemopoietic growth factor cDNA in a factor-dependent cell line results in autonomous growth and tumourigenicity. Cell 33:153-159

Mann R, Mulligan RC, Baltimore D (1983) Construction of a retrovirus packaging mutant and its use to produce helper-free defective retrovirus. Cell 33:153-159

Metcalf D (1985) The granulocyte-macrophage colony-stimulating factors. Science 229:16-22

Oppi C, Shore SK, Reddy EP (1987) Nucleotide sequence of testis-derived c-abl cDNAs: implications for testis-specific transcription and abl oncogene activation. Proc. Natl. Acad. Sci. USA 84:8200-8204

Shaw G, Kamen R (1986) A conserved AU sequence from the 3' untranslated region of GM-CSF mRNA mediates selective mRNA degradation. Cell 46:659-667.

Shtivelman E, Lifshitz B, Gale RP, Canaani E (1985) Fused transcript of abl and bcr genes in chronic myelogenous leukaemia. Nature 315:550-554

Biological Effects of Retroviral Transfection of the Murine Interleukin-3 Gene into FDCP-Mix Cells

Elaine Spooncer, Makoto Katsuno, Ian Hampson, T Michael Dexter, Ursula Just*, Carol Stocking*, Norbert Kluge*, Wolfram Ostertag*

Paterson Institute for Cancer Research, Christie Hospital and Holt Radium Institute, Wilmslow Road, Manchester, M20 9BX, UK; *Heinrich-Pette Institute, 2000 Hamburg 20, Germany

INTRODUCTION

Several genetic changes are believed to be necessary to convert normal haemopoietic cells into leukaemic cells. These changes are associated with various biological events including immortalisation, clonal selection, changes in growth factor requirements and stromal cell dependence and changes in the balance of self-renewal and differentiation. Within the haemopoietic system, a variety of growth factors are now known to play a critical role in recruiting proliferation and development of the most primitive multipotent stem cells and the lineage-restricted progenitor cells. Some of these growth factors are biologically restricted and are able to recruit only the lineage-restricted progenitor cells (e.g. M-CSF, G-CSF and erythropoietin); others show a broader range of activities and can stimulate growth and development of multipotent stem cells and facilitate their development into several cell lineages (Dexter 1987). An example of the latter class of growth factor is Interleukin-3 (IL3). Because multipotent stem cells are the putative target cells for malignant transformation, it is clearly of importance to determine how IL3 influences the various parameters associated with the growth of normal cells and the influence (if any) that aberrant production of (or response to) this growth factor may have in leukaemic transformation. One problem with such studies, however, is that stem cells represent only about 0.01% of the marrow cell population and _direct_ analysis of the effects of growth factors is difficult to perform on these cells. To circumvent this problem, we have exploited the ability of IL3 (and more recently GM-CSF) to allow the continuing growth _in vitro_ of multipotent stem cells (FDCP-Mix), which can be readily cloned in soft agar and exhibits many of the properties of normal stem cells. As part of our studies, we have used these cells to determine the effects of induced expression of the IL3 gene (_i.e._ autocrine stimulation) transferred into the cells by a retroviral vector.

FDCP-MIX CELL LINES

The target cells chosen for retroviral transfer of the IL3 gene are a class of cell lines, FDCP-Mix (Factor Dependent Cells Paterson) (Spooncer et al 1986). These cell lines are derived from mouse long-term bone marrow cultures infected with virus carrying the avian v-_src_ oncogene. The stromal cells of v-_src_-infected long-term cultures express the pp60v-_src_ protein and become morphologically transformed, and haemopoietic cell development is profoundly altered, presumably due to alterations in the regulatory environment of the stromal cells. The developmental profile of haemopoietic cells is "inverted", i.e. there is a high concentration of primitive

Current Topics in Microbiology and Immunology, Vol. 149

haemopoietic cells with an unusually high capacity to express self-renewal and an almost complete block in differentiation, resulting in the production of only few mature cells (Boettiger et al 1984). Haemopoietic cell lines can readily be established and cloned from src-infected long-term cultures. The cell lines are absolutely dependent on IL3 for survival, and termed FDCP-Mix cells. Of major importance is that, unlike the stromal cells from the v-src-infected cultures the FDCP-Mix cells do not have integrated src virus and do not, therefore, express high levels of pp60v-src protein. They do, however, produce the ecotropic "helper" virus used to facilitate v-src infection of the original cultures. When grown in suspension cultures with IL3 and horse serum the cells maintain > 90% blast cell morphology. They have a high clonogenic capacity (2.5 - 25% clonogenic cells), are diploid and non-leukaemic. A most interesting characteristic of FDCP-Mix cells is their ability to differentiate into most myeloid cell types in response to culture conditions that promote differentiation of normal primitive haemopoietic cells in vitro e.g. semi-solid CFC-Mix assay. Furthermore, when seeded onto inductive haemopoietic stroma the FDCP-Mix cells can attach, proliferate and differentiate, in the same way as normal primitive haemopoietic cells (Spooncer et al 1986). FDCP-Mix cells therefore provide a model for analysing the effects of induced IL3 expression on growth factor requirements, stromal cell interaction, differentiation potential and leukemogenesis.

RETROVIRAL INFECTION OF FDCP-MIX CELLS WITH THE IL3 GENE

Since the FDCP-Mix cells are constitutive producers of the ecotropic helper virus used in the original long-term culture infections, (i.e. surface receptors for ecotropic virus are therefore blocked) an amphotropic virus was constructed for the retroviral transfer of the IL3 gene into the cells. A cDNA clone of IL3 (provided by N Gough, Melbourne) was subcloned into the murine myelo-proliferative sarcoma virus-based vector carrying a dominant selectable marker conferring resistance to G418 (MPSV M3neo^r). This vector was transfected into the amphotropic helper cell line, PA317 to generate a cell line producing infectious amphotropic pseudotypes carrying the IL3 and neo^r gene (M3MuV). PA317 cells producing amphotropic pseudotypes carrying the M3neo^r gene only were used for control infections. Producer cell lines with titres between 10^3 - 10^5 GTU for the M3MuV virus and 10^5 - 10^8 GTU for the M3neo^r virus, with intact proviral genomes, were used for infecting FDCP-Mix cells (Laker et al 1987, Stocking et al 1985).

Sub-confluent cultures of the virus producer cells were irradiated with 20Gy from a Cobalt-60 source to prevent subsequent contamination of the FDCP-Mix cells with the vigorous PA317. FDCP-Mix cells were harvested during the logarithmic phase of growth and seeded onto producer cells at 10^5 cells/ml in Iscove's medium supplemented with 20% v/v horse serum and IL3 (complete growth medium). Non-adherent and loosely adherent FDCP-Mix cells were harvested from the co-cultures 48h later. Clumps of dead and dying producer cells were allowed to sediment at 1g for 5 minutes and the FDCP-Mix cells were washed and resuspended in complete growth medium supplemented with G418 (1 mg/ml) at 3 x 10^5 cells/ml. During the following 7 days extensive cell death occurred and live cells were separated using a buoyant density gradient of 1.080 g/ml. Surviving cells were expanded and cloned in semi-solid agar in the presence of IL3 and G418. Individual clones were picked from agar cultures and transferred to liquid culture. FDCP-Mix cells infected with the M3neo^r virus were termed FDCP-Mix-neo^r and those infected with the M3MuV virus (which were subsequently shown to be able to proliferative in the absence of added IL3) were termed FICP-Mix-IL3 (i.e. Factor Independent).

Integration of the M3MuV Virus in FDCP-Mix Cells

The viral insertion sites were determined in 3 separate clones of FICP-Mix-IL3 cells by Southern analysis. The DNA was EcoRI, Sac I and Hind III restricted and probed with neomycin and IL3 cDNA. Each clone exhibited a unique insertion site. In the construction of the MPSV-based M3MuV vector the IL3 cDNA was cloned into the RI site (Laker et al 1987). Southern analysis of EcoRI restricted DNA isolated from FDCP-Mix-neo^r and two clones of FICP-Mix-IL3 showed all 3 contained the endogenous IL3 gene. Only the two M3MuV-infected clones also contained the retrovirally-derived EcoRI restricted IL3 fragment. This confirmed that the retroviral vector carrying the intact IL3 gene was integrated into the FDCP-Mix cells.

BIOLOGICAL CHARACTERISTICS OF FICP-MIX-IL3

Growth Factor Dependence

In the absence of IL3, FDCP-Mix cells and FDCP-Mix-neo^r died within 48h regardless of the initial cell concentration. However, the cell lines infected with the M3MuV virus could survive and proliferate in the absence of IL3 (Fig 1).

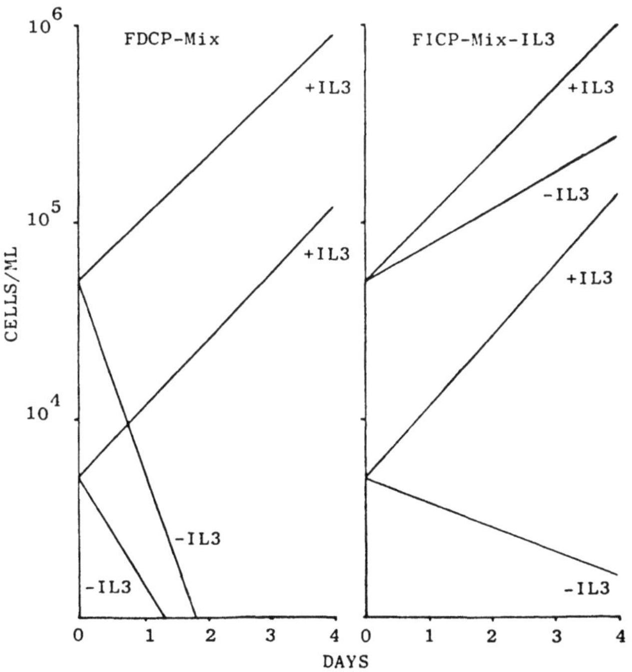

Fig. 1. Growth curves of FDCP-Mix and FICP-Mix-IL3

Survival in the absence of growth factor was cell density-dependent in that below a certain cell concentration (5 x 10^3 cells/ml) FICP-Mix-IL3 cells could not survive in the absence of IL3. Furthermore, addition of exogeneous IL3 to cultures of these cells enhanced the growth rate of the cells. These results suggest that the FICP-Mix-IL3 cells produce IL3 in rate-limiting quantity for the growth of the cells. This suggestion was supported by quantitation of IL3 secreted into the growth medium by the cells. Conditioned medium harvested from high-density cell cultures was assayed for IL3 activity using an IL3-dependent indicater cell line. The FICP-Mix-IL3 cells produced between 4 and 50 units of IL3 per ml, whereas (in the same assay) WEH1-3BD$^-$ cells produced 500 units of IL3 per ml (Bazill et al 1983).

The data suggest that, at high cell density, IL3 independence is mediated by an autocrine mechanism. To determine if this autocrine growth represents external stimulation of cells via receptor occupation by the endogenously produced IL3, one clone of M3MuV virus infected cells was treated with neutralising antisera to IL3. Figure 2 clearly shows that growth is inhibited by antiserum i.e. the growth of FICP-Mix-IL3 occurs via an autocrine mechanism involving secretion of IL3 and subsequent receptor mediated stimulation.

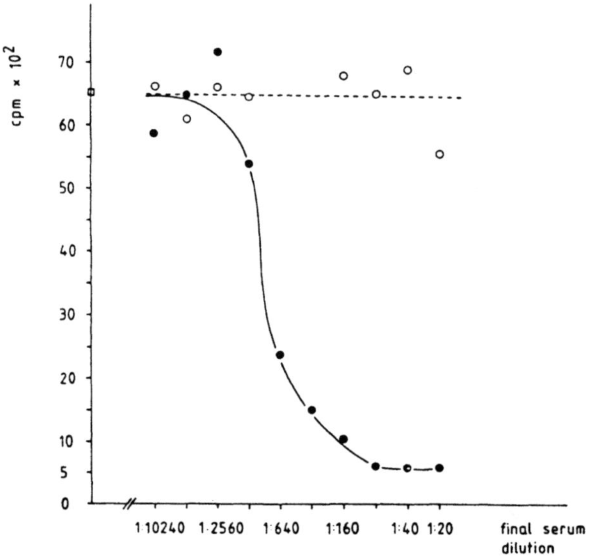

Fig 2. Growth Inhibition of FICP-Mix-IL3 Cells by anti-IL3 Antiserum.

● growth medium with rabbit anti-IL3 antiserum
O growth medium with preimmuneserum
□ growth medium alone

30h after initiation of cultures in the above conditions 0.5 µCi ^{3}H-thymidine was added for 14h. Cells were harvested onto filters and counted.

Differentiation Potential

The differentiation potential of FICP-Mix-IL3 cells was investigated using the CFC-Mix semi-solid agar assay in the presence of fetal calf serum, bovine serum albumin, IL3 and erythropoietin (Spooncer et al 1986). In five separate experiments 30 colonies from each group were pooled and disaggregated in groups of five colonies. Cytospin preparations were made from each group and stained with May-Grunwald Giemsa and dimethyl benzidine. More than 100 cells were scored from each group. The results in Table 1 show that under these conditions the concentration of clonogenic cells is not altered by the M3MuV virus and that the infected cells are still able to undergo granulocytic differentiation. Erythroid cells were consistently absent from the colonies derived from the FICP-Mix-IL3 cells although the cells infected with neo^r alone were not altered in their erythroid potential. Thus, the introduction of the IL3 gene into FDCP-Mix cells does not block differentiation, but did appear to restrict erythroid maturation *in vitro*.

Table 1 Differentiation of FDCP-Mix Cells In Vitro

	PE%	bl/eg	lg	mono	E'bl/BZ
FDCP-Mix	5.5	14	53	12	21
FDCP-Mix-neo^r	5.0	10	58	12	20
FICP-Mix-IL3	6.2	22	51	27	0

PE% - plating efficiency (number of colonies per 100 cells);
bl/eg - primitive blast cells, promyelocytes and myelocytes;
lg - metamyelocytes and neutrophils;
mono - large mononuclear cells;
E'bl/BZ - erythroblasts and benzidine positive cells (haemoglobin+ve);
Standard error less that ± 10%.

Interaction of FICP-Mix-IL3 Cells with Haemopoietic Stroma

FICP-Mix-IL3 cells infected with the M3MuV virus retain the ability to attach and grow on stromal cell layers in the absence of added IL3. However, there is a distinct difference between the kinetics of attachment and growth of these cells compared to the parental FDCP-Mix cells in that fewer cells attach, they take longer to form foci within the stroma and the foci do not grow so large. Furthermore, within 7 days of seeding FDCP-Mix cells onto a stromal cell layer, 75-90% of the cells produced are mature granulocytes (Spooncer et al 1986), yet it takes 2-3 weeks for mature cells to emerge when FICP-Mix-IL3 are cultured with stromal cells. The percentage of mature cells is only 10-60%, and many primitive cells persist. When cultured in the presence of stroma, therefore, the FICP-Mix-IL3 cells maintain a higher probability of self-renewal than the parent FDCP-Mix cells. It is not clear whether this alteration in the response to stromal cells is the result of the secretion of IL3 into the growth medium by the FICP-Mix-IL3 cells or whether it is an intrinsic alteration in the ability of the cells to attach and subsequently respond to stromal cell regulatory signals.

IN VIVO ADMINISTRATION OF FICP-MIX-IL3 CELLS

Non-infected FDCP-Mix cells do form spleen colonies in irradiated mice but this capacity is restricted to early isolates of the cell line. The nature of the spleen colonies is a puzzle as we have shown many times that FDCP-Mix cells do not rescue lethally irradiated mice from haemopoietic failure. Thus it seems the cells can not re-establish haemopoietic function *in vivo* to the extent that mice will survive, nor do the FDCP-Mix cells induce any disease in normal or irradiated mice when up to 10^7 cells are infected (Spooncer et al 1986).

Low numbers (5×10^4 - 5×10^5) of FICP-Mix-IL3 cells were injected into potentially lethally irradiated mice and some of the mice were killed 10 days later. Colonies of cells were evident on the spleens of the mice and karyotypic analysis showed that the injected (male) cells were indeed proliferating in the bone marrow and spleen of the irradiated (female) mice. Evidently the FICP-Mix-IL3 cells could proliferate and grow in irradiated recipients, at least in the short term. The injected cells did not promote survival of the irradiated mice which, if not killed for analysis, were all dead within 3 weeks of injection. Morphological analysis of the spleens and of these mice 10d after injection of the IL3-infected cells showed predominantly erythroid development (85-95% of cells) the remainder comprising of blast cells, early and late granulocytes, lymphoid cells and eosinophils i.e. a similar picture to that seen in normal regenerating spleen. It is not clear if these mice died due to the inability of the injected cells to reconstitute functional haemopoiesis or whether the injected cells actively contributed to the cause of death.

FICP-Mix-IL3 cells were then injected into immunosuppressed (sub-lethally irradiated) recipient mice. Within 3 months of receiving an inoculum of 5×10^6 cells the mice exhibited haematological abnormalities and morbidity which subsequently led to their death with 6 months. The main features observed in the mice were massive splenomegally, a dramatic increase in circulating leukocytes, a severe anaemia and slight bone marrow aplasia (Table 2). Morphological analysis of spleen, peripheral blood and bone marrow indicated that FDCP-Mix-IL3 cells produce a chronic myeloid leukaemia-like (CML) disorder (Table 3).

Table 2 In Vivo Administration of FDCP-Mix and FICP-Mix-IL3 Cells

	Cells injected (5×10^6/mouse)	
	FDCP-Mix and FDCP-Mix-neo^r	FICP-Mix-IL3
Incidence of "CML"	$^0/_{50}$	$^{50}/_{50}$
Spleen Weight (mg, range)	70 - 120	530 - 1280
Blood Counts ($\times 10^{-3}$/mm^3, range)	3 - 7	29 - 276
Femur Cellularity ($\times 10^7$, range)	1.2 - 2.3	0.4 - 1.1
Haematocrit	39 - 44	19 - 36

Table 3 Differential Analysis of Haemopoietic Tissue from Sublethally Irradiated Mice Injected with FDCP-Mix-neo^r and FDCP-Mix-IL3

Cells injected	Tissue[a]	bl[b]	eg	lg	ly	ery	other
FDCP-Mix-neo^r	PB	0	0	25	73	0	2
	SP	0	0	4	93	1	2
	BM	2	23	39	8	24	4
FDCP-Mix-IL3	PB	2	14	75	4	2	3
	SP	5	21	38	15	18	3
	BM	3	9	76	4	16	2

[a] PB - peripheral blood; SP - spleen; BM- bone marrow.
[b] bl, eg, lg - as in Table 1; ly - lymphoid; ery - nucleated erythroid cells; other - macrophage, megakaryocyte, eosinophil, basophil/mast cells.
10 mice were examined 3-4 months after cells were injected. The data are from one mouse in each group and are representative. In two mice eosinophilia (PB 18%, SP 13% and BM 7%) was observed.

The origin of cells growing in spleen, peripheral blood and bone marrow of these mice was analysed by Southern analysis using a Y-chromosome DNA probe (80/YB) (Avner et al 1987). This probe can detect a male/female mixture down to a male component of only 0.5%. Results showed no male cells detectable indicating that the disease was in fact largely of host (female) origin and not therefore the result of the growth of the injected (male) cells. Thus, in recipient mice where haemopoiesis is totally ablated M3MuV-infected cells can grow and proliferate at least for 2 weeks whereas in partially ablated mice infected with these cells the origin of the resultant disease is predominantly recipient cells. The helper virus which is constitutively produced by the FDCP-Mix cells permits continued production of the M3MuV virus following injection of the cells. This virus, therefore has the potential to infect the cells of the recipient animal. Nevertheless, injection of highly concentrated M3MuV virus into mice does not result in any disease. We speculate that injecting the virus in association with cells that can persist in the recipient (at least in the short term) and may home specifically to haemopoietic organs provides a mechanism for targeting the virus to particular regions and may produce infectious centres subsequently leading to recruitment of host cells and the onset of disease.

The production of IL3 by the IL3-infected cells in vivo may also play a role in the development of the CML-like disorder. Indeed, Northern analysis of spleen cells from these mice probed with IL3 cDNA confirmed the presence of IL3 transcripts. No IL3 transcript was detected in normal spleen cells.

In vivo the effects of FICP-Mix-IL3 infected cells may be a combination of virus production and targeting and IL3 production; at present we have not determined the mechanism underlying the emergence of the CML-like disorder.

DISCUSSION

FDCP-Mix cells are (unlike normal stem cells) immortalised in the presence of IL3: this immortalisation requires IL3 but presumably includes also a degree of genetic re-programming intrinsic to the FDCP-Mix which allows them to self-renew (rather than differentiate) in IL3. This re-programming sets them apart from normal stem cells. However, the programming is by no means immutable: the probability of self-renewal versus differentiation is also determined by other external influences such as serum components or marrow stromal cells (Spooncer et al 1986). The introduction of the IL3-gene into the cells leads to changes in the cells that can be well characterised *in vitro* i.e. the self-stimulation of growth ("intrinsic" immortalisation) which allows the cells to grow continuously in the absence of added IL3; a moderation of the differentiation potential of the cells such that granulocytic potential is virtually unchanged yet erythroid development is very restricted *in vitro*; and modulation in the interaction of FICP-Mix-IL3 cells with haemopoietic stroma.

How the *in vitro* changes in the characteristics of the FICP-Mix-IL3 cells correlate with their ability to induce a CML-like disorder *in vivo* is difficult to assess due to the multiple factors that may be involved in the disease development. The development of the FICP-Mix-IL3 cells and the progression from factor-dependence to factor-independence has so far required at least two steps. The introduction of further genes into these cells (growth factors or oncogenes) or insertional mutagenesis should permit the examination of the process of differentiation and the conversion of growth factor-independent but differentiation inducible cells into cells which are blocked in differentiation.

REFERENCES

Avner P, Bishop C, Amar L, Cambrou J, Hatat D, Arnaud, Mattei M-G (1987) Mapping the mouse X chromosome: possible symmetry in the location of a family of sequences on the mouse X and Y chromosomes. Development 101 (Supplement): 107-116

Bazill GW, Haynes M, Garland J, Dexter TM (1983) Characterisation and partial purification of a haemopoietic cell growth factor in WEH1-3 cell conditioned medium. 210: 747-759

Boettiger D, Anderson S, Dexter TM (1984) Effect of *src* infection on long-term marrow cultures: Increased self renewal of hemopoietic progenitor cells without leukaemia. Cell 36: 763-773

Dexter TM (1987) Stem cells in normal growth and diseases. British Medical J. 295: 1192-1194

Laker C, Stocking C, Bergholz U, Hess W, DeLamarter JF, Ostertag W (1987) Autocrine stimulation after transfer of the granulocyte/macrophage colony stimulating factor gene and autonomous growth are distinct but interdependent steps in the oncogenic pathway. Proc Natl Acad Sci USA 84: 8458-8462

Spooncer E, Boettiger D, Dexter TM (1985) Continuous *in vitro* generation of multipotential stem cell clones from *src*-infected cultures. Nature 310: 228-230

Spooncer E, Heyworth CM, Dunn A, Dexter TM (1986) Self-renewal and differentiation of Interleukin-3-dependent multipotent stem cells are modulated by stromal cells and serum factors. Differentiation 31: 111-118

Stocking C, Kollek R, Bergholz U, Ostertag W (1985) Long terminal repeat sequences impart haematopoietic transformation properties to the myeloproliferative sarcoma virus. Proc Natl Acad Sci USA 82: 5746-5750

Conversion of Factor-Dependent Myeloid Cells to Factor Independence: Autocrine Stimulation is Not Coincident with Tumorigenicity

C. Stocking, M. Kawai*, C. Laker, C. Löliger[1], N, Kluge, K. Klingler[2], and W. Ostertag

Heinrich-Pette-Institut für Experimentelle Virologie und Immunologie an der Universität Hamburg, 2000 Hamburg 20, FRG
*Dept. of Microbiolgy, Aichi Medical University, Nagakute-cho, Aichi 480-11, Japan

INTRODUCTION

Release from normal growth requirements has long been hypothesized as an initial step in malignant progression (Holley, 1976). All cells of the myeloid lineage, from early progenitors to mature blood cells, are under the immediate control of certain growth factors that support their survival, proliferation, differentiation, and functional activation. Four of these growth factors have been characterized in in vitro culture systems for both mouse and human (for reviews see Metcalf, 1985 and Clark and Kamen, 1987). In vitro analysis of the mechanisms that may lead to disruption of the normal controls governing proliferation and differentiation is made feasible by the availability of established hematopoietic cell lines that are dependent on one or several of these factors for survival and proliferation and, in some cases, are still responsive to differentiation stimuli (Greenberger et al., 1980; Dexter et al., 1980). We present here evidence that support the hypothesis that aberrant expression of a growth factor and subsequent stimulation by an autocrine mechanism may play a pivotal role in the initial stages of malignant progression, however, tumorigenesis is not coincident with autocrine stimulation.

ISOLATION OF FACTOR-INDEPENDENT MUTANTS

Previous attempts to determine the mechanism by which hematopoietic cells may escape normal growth controls have usually involved the introduction and expression of a known oncogene or growth factor in a cell line followed by assessment of factor-dependent growth and tumorigenicty (Adkins et al., 1984; Cook et al., 1985; Lang et al., 1985; Pierce et al., 1985). An alternate approach is to analyze spontaneous factor-dependent mutants. We first established the frequency of mutations that lead to factor-independent growth in a hematopoietic cell line. The promyelocytic cell line D35 was established after in vitro infection of a long-term bone marrow culture with a Friend spleen focus forming virus (F-SFFV) and Rauscher murine leukemia virus (R-MuLV) complex (Greenberger et al., 1980). D35 cells require either the multi-lineage colony stimulating factor, interleukin 3 (IL3), or the granulocyte-macrophage colony stimulating factor (GM-CSF) for cell growth. When required factor was removed by dilution over a period of two to three weeks, factor-independent

[1]Present Address: Dept. of Microbiology, University of Southern California, Los Angeles, CA 90000, USA
[2]Present Address: Walter and Eliza Hall Institute of Medical Research, P.O. Royal Melbourne Hospital, Victoria 3050, Australia

Current Topics in Microbiology and Immunology, Vol. 149

mutants could be isolated at a frequency of 2.4 $x10^{-7}$ (Stocking et al., 1988, Kawai et al., submitted). This frequency was not altered when the D35 line was recloned to insure that the mutants isolated were not part of a sub-population of cells within the parental line. Cells growing in media without factor after three weeks were cloned in methylcellulose and designated Dind for D35 factor independent. Thirteen Dind mutants were further characterized to elucidate possible mechanisms leading to factor-independent growth.

Majority of Mutants Release Growth Factor

To determine if any of the Dind mutants had acquired factor-dependent growth via "autocrine stimulation"--in which a cell's growth is stimulated by factor released by the cell itself (DeLarco and Todaro, 1978)--, conditioned media (CM) of eleven mutants were assayed for mitogenic activity on the parental D35 cell line. All Dind mutants, except Dind2 and Dind3, released an activity that supported normal growth of the D35 cell line. Limited growth of D35 cells was obtained with Dind2 supernatant, and a subpopulation of D35 cells could be cloned that responded to Dind2 CM almost as well as growth of the original D35 cells when stimulated with Dind1 CM.

To characterize the factor released by the Dind mutants, CM was used to stimulate four different indicator lines. Six mutants, Dind1, 4, 5, 9, 10, 13, 14, and 15, release a factor that stimulated only cell lines responsive to both growth factors but not cell lines responsive to IL3 alone and thus most likely secrete GM-CSF. Three mutants, Dind6, 7, and 8, release an activity that stimulated all indicator lines, including those with a strict requirement for IL3. Hybridization of total RNA isolated from Dind mutants with specific probes confirmed that nine of the mutants expressed GM-CSF and three expressed IL-3. No IL3 or GM-CSF transcripts could be detected in Dind2 or Dind3. Results are summarized in Table 1.

Table 1. Summary of D35 Factor-Independent Mutants

	Growth Stimulation		Northern Analysis					Southern Analysis
	D35[a] FDC-P1	SUtA[b] FDC-P2	IL3	G/M[c]	G[c]	M[c]	IL4	
D35	-	-	-	-	-	-	+	
Dind1	+++	-	-	++	-	-	+	rearranged GM (3')
Dind2	(+)	-	-	-	-	-	+	normal
Dind3	-	-	-	-	-	-	+	normal
Dind4	+++	-	-	+++	-	-	+	rearranged GM (5')
Dind5	+++	-	-	+++	-	-	+	rearranged GM (5')
Dind6	+++	+++	+	-	nt[d]	nt	nt	normal
Dind7	+++	++	++	-	nt	nt	nt	rearranged IL3 (5')
Dind8	+++	++	+++	-	nt	nt	nt	rearranged IL3 (5')
Dind9	+++	-	-	+++	nt	nt	nt	rearranged GM (5')
Dind10	+++	-	-	+++	nt	nt	nt	normal
Dind13	+++	-	-	nt	nt	nt	nt	
Dind14	+++	-	-	nt	nt	nt	nt	
Dind15	+++	-	-	+++	nt	nt	nt	normal

[a] Cells are responsive to either IL3 or GM-CSF
[b] Cells are only responsive to IL3
[c] Granulocyte and/or Macrophage colony stimulating factors
[d] nt; not tested

Activation of Growth Factor Allele by Retrotransposons

Aberrant growth factor secretion can be a consequence of either mutations within the growth factor gene itself or by activation or suppression of a second cellular gene (e.g. proto-oncogene) that may regulate the growth factor gene. Rearrangements of one of the corresponding alleles was detected in four out of six Dind mutants (Dindl, 4, 5, and 9) which expressed GM-CSF and two out of three Dind mutants (Dind7 and 8) which expressed IL3. Analysis of the four Dind mutants with obvious structural alterations in one of the GM-CSF alleles revealed that either a retrovirus or other retrotransposon had integrated near to or in the transcribed region. In Dind4, 5, and 9, the provirus of one of the two viruses that had been used to establish the parental D35 line had integrated between 250 and 700bp upstream of the cap site. In the case of Dindl, an intracisternal A particle (IAP) genome was integrated downstream of the coding region but within the transcribed gene. Fig. 1 depicts the insertions in the GM-CSF locus characterized by molecular cloning and Southern analysis (Stocking et al., 1988.)

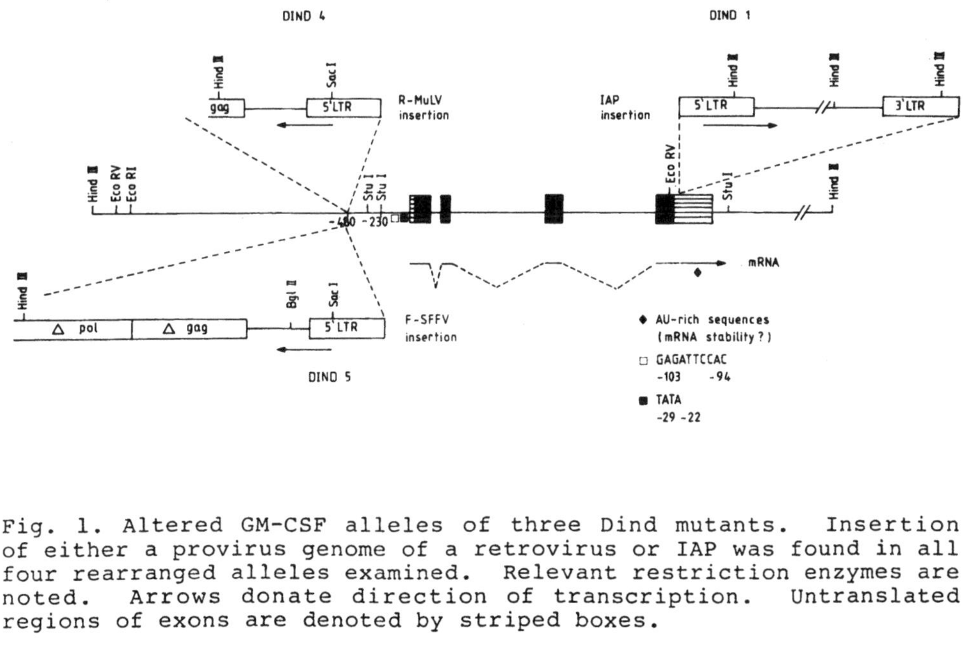

Fig. 1. Altered GM-CSF alleles of three Dind mutants. Insertion of either a provirus genome of a retrovirus or IAP was found in all four rearranged alleles examined. Relevant restriction enzymes are noted. Arrows donate direction of transcription. Untranslated regions of exons are denoted by striped boxes.

It was demonstrated that the rearranged alleles were the transcriptionally active alleles by expression assays of cloned DNA of the wild-type and mutated allele in Dind mutants where insertion had occurred 5'of the gene. RNAse protection assays of the GM-CSF transcript where integration had occurred in the 3' non-coding, but transcribed, region confirmed active transcription from the altered allele in Dindl. It is of interest to note that GM-CSF transcripts in Dindl have lost an AU-rich region, often found in mRNAs of the transiently expressed growth factor genes and postulated to impart reduced RNA stability in eukaryotic transcripts (Shaw and Kamen,

1986), due to insertion of the IAP exactly seven bp downstream of the normal GM-CSF termination codon. Experiments are in progress to determine if stability of the GM-CSF RNA has been altered in this cell line, thereby allowing sufficient levels of the mRNA for growth stimulation when transcription is only weakly promoted.

Non-linear Plating Efficiency and the Presence of Active GM-CSF Receptors Supports Autocrine Stimulation Model

The autogenous production of growth factor by the D35 variants could have been either a causal event that resulted in the factor-independent growth of the D35 variants or, alternatively, a fortuitous secondary event that was independent of the acquired autonomy. To exclude the latter possibility, the plating efficiency as a function of cell densitiy was determined for an early and late passage of Dind1 cells (Kawai _et al._, submitted; Fig. 2). Clonability was compared in the presence and absence of WEHI-3B supernatant (WEHI-CM), used as a source of IL3. In the presence of added growth factor the relationship of number of cells plated and number of colonies was linear; however, in medium alone the relationship was non-linear, with a higher plating efficiency occurring when higher numbers of cells from the early passage were plated. These results support the hypothesis that factor-independent growth was acquired by autocrine stimulation. Later passages of Dind1 cells, however, cloned equally well in the presence or absence of an added source of growth factor, indicating that subsequent events have occured that have resulted in true growth autonomy.

The presence of GM-CSF-specific receptors was determined by ^{125}I-labeled recombinant GM-CSF (Biogen) binding to D35 cells and four Dind mutants (Kawai _et al._, submitted). Specific binding was detected in both Dind1 _and_ Dind4 mutants, however, at reduced levels: 30-50% and 10-25% for Dind1 and Dind4, respectively, of the parental D35 line. This reduction most likely reflects competitive blocking of the receptors by autocrine-secreted GM-CSF and would support the hypothesis that the secreted GM-CSF stimulates receptors found on the cell surface. No receptors were detected on Dind2 or Dind3. Whether this is directly correlated with the mechanism by which these mutants have obtained factor independence or reflects a pre-existing population of D35 cells that are not responsive to GM-CSF cannot be ascertained at present.

Is Autocrine Stimulation Coexistent with Tumorigenicity?

Schrader and Crapper (1983) and Lang _et al._ (1985) have shown that tumorigenicty as measured by tumor formation in nude mice may be a property of hematopoietic cells that have acquired factor independent growth by autonomous CSF production. Mice inoculated with 10^{-7} cells each from either the Dind1 or Dind4 cell line developed ascitic tumors within three to six weeks, whereas D35 cell did not elicit tumor formation until three to four months following injection (most likely arising as a consequence of leukemia induced by the Friend virus complex released from the D35 cells) (Kawai _et al._, submitted). Tumors were determined to be of donor origin by use of H-2 and isoenzyme markers. Although these results support a correlation between autocrine stimulation and tumorigenicity, it could not be excluded that tumor formation was due to cells present in the Dind1 or Dind4 population that had acquired a secondary alteration, as demonstrated in the shift in cloning efficiency when the cells were maintained for extended periods in tissue culture.

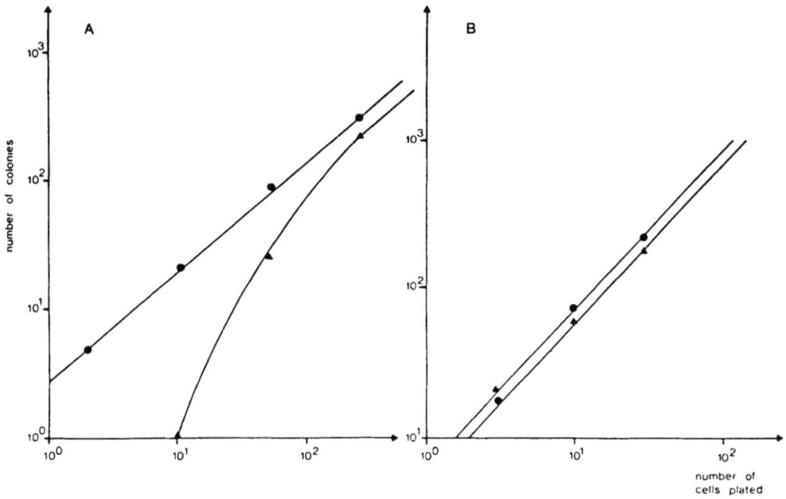

Fig. 2. Clonability of Dindl cells in the presence (●) or absence (▲) of added growth factor. Dindl cells, maintained for two weeks (panel A) or more than three months (panel B) after cloning were recloned in medium with 0.9% methyl cellulose.

EXPRESSION OF GROWTH FACTOR GENES BY RETROVIRAL VECTORS RESULTS IN AUTOCRINE STIMULATION

Retroviral vectors containing the cDNA clones for either GM-CSF or IL3 were used to infect two other promyelocytic cell lines, FDC-P1 and FDC-P2 (Dexter et al., 1980), to address several questions raised by the results of the Dind analysis: 1) Does autogenous production of a required factor lead to factor dependent growth in one step and is the action of the autogenous factor specific for cells which express the appropriate receptor?; 2) Is the acquistion of factor independent growth by autocrine stimulation coincident with tumorigenesis?; 3) Can autonomous growth in vitro (e.g. cell-density independent cloning) be correlated with tumorigenicity?

Two types of vectors were constructed based on the myeloproliferative sarcoma virus (MPSV) and carrying the Tn5 neomycin resistance gene (neo^R) that confers resistance to the aminoglycoside G418 in eukaryotes (Fig. 3). MPSV has been shown to contain unique LTR sequences which allow efficient transcriptional activity in both hematopoietic and embryonic stem cells (Stocking et al., 1985; Hilberg et al., 1987.) The M3neo series of vectors is designed to give relatively low expression levels of the introduced gene, whereas the M5neo expresses relatively high levels of the introduced gene. Up to a one hundred fold difference of GM-CSF production was observed between M3 GMV and M5 GMV (Laker et al., 1987).

Immediately after a 24-hour infection period, FDC-P1 and FDC-P2 cells were cloned at different cells densities in methylcellulose either in the presence of WEHI-CM and G418 or, alternatively, in the absence of any added stimulating factor. Infection of either

FDC-P1 or FDC-P2 cells with either of the two IL3 constructs (M3 MuV or M5 MuV) resulted in colony formation in the absense of WEHI-CM at high cell density (Laker *et al.*, submitted). The two GMV constructs induced colony formation in the absence of added factor only in FDC-P1 cells (Laker *et al.*, 1987). This is consistent with the hypothesis that autogenous factor stimulates growth by acting directly with its cognate receptor; both FDC-P1 and FDC-P2 exhibit IL3-specific receptors, but only FDC-P1 express GM-CSF receptors on its cell surface.

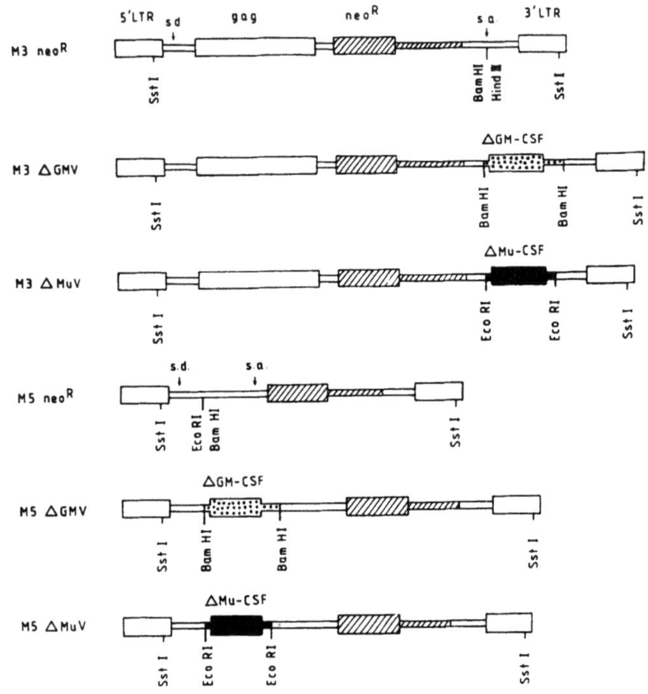

Fig. 3. MPSV-based vectors carrying the cDNAs for either GM-CSF or IL3 (Multi-CSF). Construction of vectors is described in Laker *et al.* (1987) and cDNA clones were kindly provided by N. Gough (Melbourne). Abbreviations used: LTR, long terminal repeats; s.d., splice donor consensus sequence; s.a., splice acceptor consensus sequence.

Initial cloning after infection of either IL3 and GM vectors was cell-density dependent, as demonstrated with the early passage Dindl cells. Indeed, the dependency on cell density was particularly striking with the M3 constructs in which much lower levels of factor was expressed. In addition, proliferation of GMV-infected FDC-P1 cells could be inhibited with GM-CSF antiserum (Fig. 4). Both results support a mechanism of autocrine stimulation in which externally presented receptors are activated by autogenous factor.

Secondary Event(s) Lead to Autonomous Growth

Infected FDC-P1 or FDC-P2 clones growing under minus WEHI-CM conditions were isolated and grown in plus WEHI-CM conditions for various time points and recloned as described previously. As observed in late passage Dindl cells, a shift to true autonomous growth (e.g. cell-density independence) was observed. The rate at which the shift occurred was found to be correlated with the amount of factor secreted by the individual clones. Thus M3 MuV- or M3 GM-infected clones shifted at a much lower rate. Interestingly, the proliferation of clones that exhibited autonomous growth properties could no longer be blocked by factor-specific antibody. An example of such a clone is shown in Fig. 4 (Laker et al., 1987). The irreversibility of this shift indicates the occurrence of a secondary genetic mutation. Although the nature of the second event is unknown, mutations in a receptor gene or mutations in any of the other genes involved in signal transmission may explain the abrogration of the requirement for external stimulation.

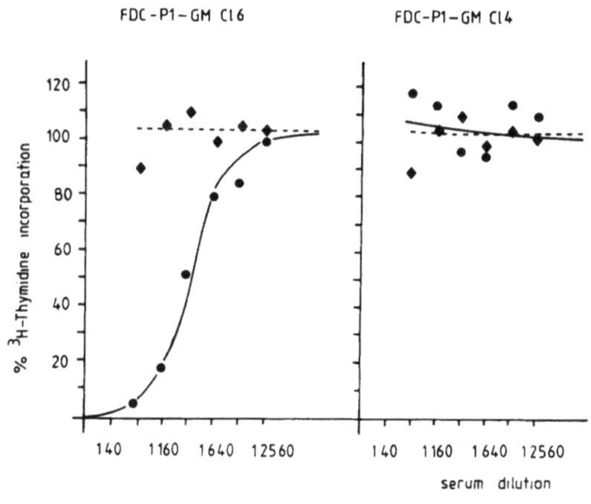

Fig. 4. Proliferation response of M3-GMV infected FDC-P1 cells after treatment with GM-CSF antiserum. Cells were treated for 48 hr with serial dilution of rabbit anti-mouse GM-CSF serum (●) or rabbit normal serum (◆) as control. Cell proliferation was assayed by (3H)thymidine incorporation. Typical non-autonomous and autonomous clones (cl 6 and cl4, respectively) are shown.

AUTONOMOUS GROWTH AND TUMORIGENICITY ARE CORRELATED

M3 MuV-infected FDC-P2 clones representative for each of the two types (i.e. factor independent but not autonomous or, alternatively, completely autonomous as judged by cloning efficiency in the absence of added factor) were used to inoculate a series of syngeneic mice. Mice injected with autonomous cells showed tumor formation after four weeks with an average tumor weight of 0.5 g; six weeks after injection average tumor weight was more than 2.5g.

In contrast to these results, mice infected with non-autonomous clones induced tumors with an average weight of 0.1g first appearing between four and six weeks after injection (Laker *et al.*, submitted). Results are depicted in Fig. 5. These data support the hypothesis that autonomous growth as defined *in vitro* could be correlated with tumorigenicity *in vivo*. It was thus of interest to evaluate the linearity of cloning efficiency as a function of cell density for cells isolated from tumors induced by both types of cells. As expected, tumors induced by autonomous clones gave rise to cells with the same growth properties; however, tumors derived from non-autonomous clones contained cells of both types. It cannot be excluded that the autonomous cells within these tumors supported the tumorigenic growth of non-autonomous cells.

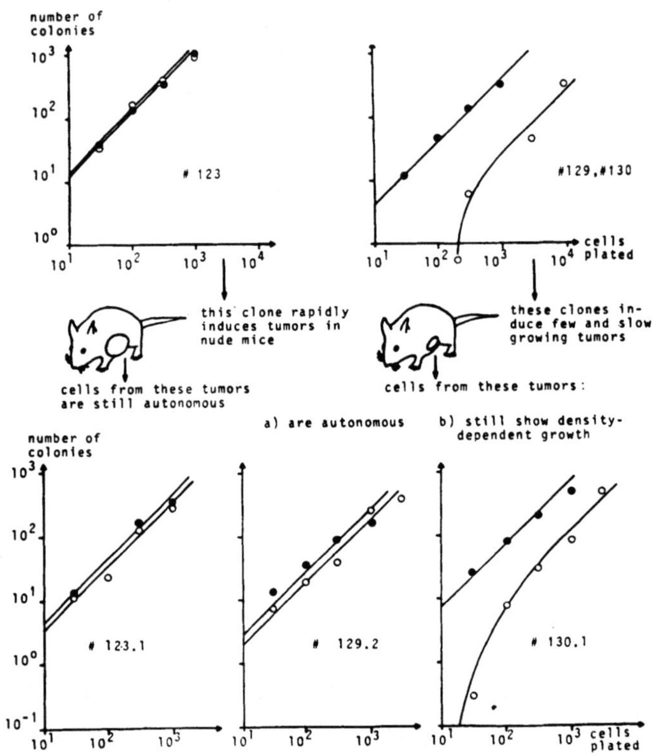

Fig. 5. Cloning efficiency as a function of cell density either in the presence of WEHI-CM (●) or in the absence of added growth factor (O). Representative clones for each type of growth property were used to infect syngeneic mice and tumor formation was monitored for up to twelve weeks (Laker *et al.*, submitted).

SUMMARY AND CONCLUSIONS

It has been postulated that the disruption of the normal hormonal regulation of blood cell formation and proliferation leads to the autonomous growth of hematopoietic progenitors or stem cells and thus to leukeamia. We have utilized established hematopoietic cell lines to establish the different mechanism by which growth autonomy is acquired. The analysis of thirteen spontaneous factor-independent mutants revealed that the majority (12/13) secreted a factor that stimulated growth of the parental cell line. Thus, autocrine stimulation may be a important mechanism by which normal growth control is disrupted. This is supported by the observation of Young and Griffin (1987) that some cells isolated from patients with acute myeloblastic leukemia (AML) autogenously produce growth factor. In the majority of Dind mutants more closely examined, growth factor gene activation was due to the juxtapostion of a retrotransposon. Although the exact nature of the involvement of human retroviruses in inducing leukemia has not been elucidated, one could envisage that altered growth factor regulation due to integration of the virus may play an important role. The existence of a second class of Dind mutants that have obtained factor-independence by a mechanism not involving factor production concurs with the acquisition of factor-independent growth in hematopoietic cells after introduction of some oncogenes. Several models have been proposed to explain how oncogenes may "short circuit" and thus activate the normal signal transduction pathway by mimicking the active receptor, transducer, or effector (Weinberg, 1985).

To investigate more closely the role of autocrine stimulation in the induction of growth autonomy and tumorigenicity, retroviral vectors expressing either GM-CSF or IL3 were introduced into factor-dependent hematopoitic cell lines. Non-linear clonability of infected cell lines in the absence of exogenous growth factor and inhibiton of proliferation by antiserum supported a model of autocrine stimulation. However, a secondary event, correlated with amount of factor released, often occured that abrogated the requirement for secreted CSF. Growth of cells in which this alteration had occured was cell-density independent and could not be blocked by antibody. It has been postulated that autogenous factor may react with its receptor intracellularly (Lang _et al._, 1985). The results presented here cannot exclude that the secondary events may allow the internal interaction of receptor and factor. Indeed, when IL3 DNA recombinants coding for an altered leader sequence which hinders efficient excretion are inserted in retroviral vectors that are used for infection, the shift to autonomy occurs at a increased rate (Laker _et al._, submitted). Tumorigenicity assays of representative clones demonstrated that autonomous growth _in vitro_ and tumorigenicity _in vivo_ were correlated. Analysis of cells derived from tumors could not exclude the hypothesis that growth autonomy is a prerequisite for tumor formation.

In conclusion, although autocrine secretion may be a general mechanism by which hematopoietic cells become factor-independent, additional, but interdependent, steps are required for tumorigenesis.

ACKNOWLEDGEMENTS

Most of this work was supported by the Deutsche Forschungsgemeinschaft and in part by the Deutsche Krebshilfe and the Fonds der Chemischen Industrie. C.S. is in the graduate studies program at the MRC Institute (London) and Brunel University. Ch.L. is a fellow of the Boehringer-Ingelheim Fonds and C.L. is a recipient of a Jung Stifftung.

REFERENCES

Adkins B, Lentz A, Graf T (1984) Autocrine growth induced by src-related oncogenes in transformed chicken myeloid cells. Cell 30:439-445
Clark S, Kamen R (1987) The human hematopoietic colony-stimulating factors. Science 236:1229-1237
Cook WD, Metcalf D, Nicola NA, Burgess AW, Walker F (1985) Malignant transformation of a growth factor-dependent myeloid cell line by Abelson virus without evidence of an autocrine mechanism. Cell 41:677-683
DeLarco JE, Todaro GJ (1978) Growth factors from murine sarcoma virus-transformed cells. Proc. Natl. Acad. Sci. USA 75:4001-4005
Dexter TM, Garland J, Scott D, Scolnick E, Metcalf D (1980) Growth of factor-dependent hemopoietic precursor cell lines. J Exp Med 152:1036-1047
Greenberger JS, Eckner RJ, Ostertag W, Colletta G, Boschetti S, Nagasawa M, Karpas A, Weichselbaum RR, Moloney WC (1980) Release of spleen focus-forming virus (SFFV) in differentiation inducible promyelocytic leukemia cell lines transformed in vitro by Friend leukemia virus. Virology 105:425-435
Hilberg F, Stocking C, Ostertag W, Grez M (1987) Functional analysis of a retroviral host-range mutant: altered long terminal repeats allow expression in embryonal carcinoma cells. Proc. Natl. Acad. Sci. USA 84:5232-5236
Holley RW (1976) Control of growth of mammalian cells in cell culture. Nature 258:487-490
Laker C, Stocking C, Bergholz U, Hess N, DeLamarter JF, Ostertag W (1987) Autocrine stimulation after transfer of the granulocyte/ macrophage colony-stimulating factor gene and autonomous growth are distinct but interdependent steps in the oncogenic pathway. Proc. Natl. Acad. Sci. USA 84:8458-8462.
Lang RA, Metcalf D, Gough N, Dunn AR, Gonda TJ (1985) Expression of a hemopoietic growth factor cDNA in a factor-dependent cell line results in autonomous growth and tumorigenicity. Cell 43:531-542
Metcalf D (1985) The granulocyte-macrophage colony-stimulating factors. Science 229:16-22
Pierce JH, DiFiore PP, Aaronson SA, Potter M, Pumphrey J, Scott A, Ihle JN (1985) Neoplastic transformation of mast cells by Abelson MuLV: abrogation of IL3 dependence by a nonautocrine mechanism. Cell 41:685-693
Schrader JW, Crapper RM (1983) Autogenous production of a hemopoietic growth factor, persisting-cell-stimulating factor, as a mechanism for transformation of bone marrow-derived cells. Proc. Natl. Acad. Sci. USA 80:6892-6896.
Shaw G, Kamen R (1986) A conserved AU sequence from the 3'untrans lated region of GM-CSF mRNA mediates selective mRNA degradation. Cell 56:659-667
Stocking C, Löliger C, Kawai M, Suciu S, Gough N, Ostertag W (1988) Identification of genes involved in growth autonomy of hematopoietic cells by analysis of factor-independent mutants. Cell 53:869-879
Stocking C, Kollek R, Bergholz U, Ostertag W (1985) Long terminal repeats impart hematopoietic transformation properties to the myeloproliferative sarcoma virus. Proc. Natl. Acad. Sci. USA 82:5746-5750
Weinberg RA (1985) The action of oncogenes in the cytoplasm and nucleus. Science 230:770-776.
Young DC, Griffin JD (1986) Autocrine secretion of GM-CSF in acute myeloblastic leukemia. Blood 68:1178-1181

V. Specific Genes Involved in Myeloid Tumorigenesis

Biosynthesis of Macrophage Colony-Stimulating Factor (CSF-1): Differential Processing of CSF-1 Precursors Suggests Alternative Mechanisms for Stimulating CSF-1 Receptors

Carl W. Rettenmier

Department of Tumor Cell Biology, St. Jude Children's Research Hospital, 332 North Lauderdale, Memphis, Tennessee 38105

INTRODUCTION

The macrophage colony-stimulating factor, M-CSF or CSF-1, is a glycosylated polypeptide homodimer required for the proliferation and differentiation of mononuclear phagocytic precursors and the survival of mature monocytes and macrophages (reviewed in Stanley et al., 1983). CSF-1 has also been reported to stimulate a variety of the immune effector functions of terminally differentiated macrophages such as phagocytosis and intracellular killing of microorganisms (Karbassi et al., 1987), tumor cell cytolysis (Wing et al., 1982; Ralph and Nakoinz, 1987), production of biocidal oxygen metabolites (Wing et al., 1985) and synthesis of plasminogen activator (Lin and Gordon 1979; Hamilton et al., 1980) as well as other cytokines including interleukin-1 (Moore et al., 1980), myeloid colony-stimulating activities (Metcalf and Nicola, 1985; Warren and Ralph, 1986), tumor necrosis factor (TNF) and interferon (Warren and Ralph, 1986). These diverse effects are mediated by binding of CSF-1 to a single high-affinity receptor on the plasma membrane of mononuclear phagocytes (Guilbert and Stanley, 1980 and 1986). The CSF-1 receptor is the c-*fms* proto-oncogene product (Sherr et al., 1985), an integral transmembrane glycoprotein that functions as a ligand-stimulated protein-tyrosine kinase (Rettenmier et al., 1985; Yeung et al., 1987; Downing et al., 1988).

In early studies many mesenchymal cells, including stromal cells of the bone marrow, were shown to produce CSF-1 which bound its receptor on mononuclear phagocytes (Tushinski et al., 1982). More recently, it has been demonstrated that peripheral blood monocytes are also induced to express the CSF-1 gene by treatment with phorbol esters, granulocyte-macrophage(GM) CSF, gamma-interferon or TNF-alpha (Horiguchi et al., 1986 and 1987; Rambaldi et al., 1987; Oster et al., 1987). This suggests that CSF-1 produced by mononuclear phagocytes at sites of inflammation may stimulate macrophage function by autocrine or paracrine mechanisms. The observation that CSF-1 transcripts are detected in blasts from about 50% of acute myelogenous leukemia (AML) patients, some of which also express the c-*fms* (CSF-1 receptor) gene, raises the possibility that autocrine production of this growth factor might also contribute to the development of these malignancies (Rambaldi et al., 1988). In addition to its role in hematopoiesis, CSF-1 synthesized by normal uterine glandular epithelial cells in response to ovarian hormones during pregnancy appears to stimulate receptor-hearing trophoblasts of the adjacent placenta (Rettenmier et al., 1986; Bartocci et al., 1986; Pollard et al., 1987).

The human gene encoding CSF-1 maps at band q33.1 on the long arm of chromosome 5 (Pettenati et al., 1987). Alternative splicing of the primary transcript generates multiple mRNA species, and biologically active cDNAs that code for two different forms of the human growth factor have been molecularly cloned (Kawasaki et al., 1985; Wong et al., 1987; Ladner et al., 1987). The deduced amino acid sequences of polypeptides encoded by these clones suggested that soluble CSF-1 is generated by proteolytic cleavage of membrane-bound precursors. Constitutive expression of the human CSF-1 products at high levels using viral vectors has permitted a direct biochemical analysis of their synthesis and processing. These studies have demonstrated that the two CSF-1 precursors differ with respect to both the sites of cleavage in the polypeptide chains and the subcellular locations where these proteolytic events take place. The differences may reflect diverse mechanisms for the stimulation of CSF-1 receptor-bearing cells by the various forms of the growth factor *in vivo*.

DIFFERENTIAL PROCESSING OF MEMBRANE-BOUND CSF-1 PRECURSORS

Multiple forms of human CSF-1 mRNA and protein

Three biologically active human CSF-1 cDNAs have been molecularly cloned (Kawasaki et al., 1985; Wong et al., 1987; Ladner et al., 1987). Nucleotide sequence analyses revealed that two distinct CSF-1 products are encoded among the various transcripts. Both primary translation products are predicted to be membrane-bound glycoproteins from which the soluble forms of the growth factor must be derived by proteolytic cleavage. A 1.6 kilobase (kb) cDNA (Kawasaki et al., 1985) specifies a 256 amino acid precursor which consists of an aminoterminal signal peptide (residues -32 to -1) for insertion of the nascent polypeptide into the membrane of the endoplasmic reticulum (ER), followed by the sequence of secreted CSF-1 (residues 1 to ca. 165), a presumptive membrane-spanning segment of hydrophobic amino acids (residues 166-188) and a short carboxylterminal tail (residues 189-224). The predicted transmembrane topology of this molecule in the ER would orient its C-terminal tail segment in the cytoplasm and its biologically active growth factor moiety within the cisternae. Thus, the N-terminal CSF-1 domain would be accessible to glycosyl transferases within the lumen of the ER for addition of asparagine(N)-linked oligosaccharides to the two canonical acceptor sequences (Asn-X-Ser/Thr).

Two independently derived cDNA clones of ca. 4 kb both encode a 554 amino acid CSF-1 precursor, which includes all of the coding sequences of the 1.6 kb cDNA product with an additional segment of 298 amino acids inserted on the aminoterminal side of the transmembrane anchor (Wong et al., 1987; Ladner et al., 1987). The block of unique coding sequences present in the 4 kb mRNAs is generated by differential splicing of exons in the primary CSF-1 gene transcript. The various human cDNAs also differ with respect to their 3' untranslated sequences. Alternative splicing of intron sequences results in differences between the 3' untranslated region of a 4 kb cDNA from a simian virus 40-transformed trophoblastic cell line (Wong et al., 1987) and that of both the 1.6 kb and 4 kb clones from a pancreatic carcinoma cell line (Kawasaki et al., 1985; Ladner et al., 1987).

The deduced structure of CSF-1 precursors encoded by the human cDNAs is diagrammed in Fig. 1. The segment corresponding to the sequence of the secreted growth factor product is indicated together with the

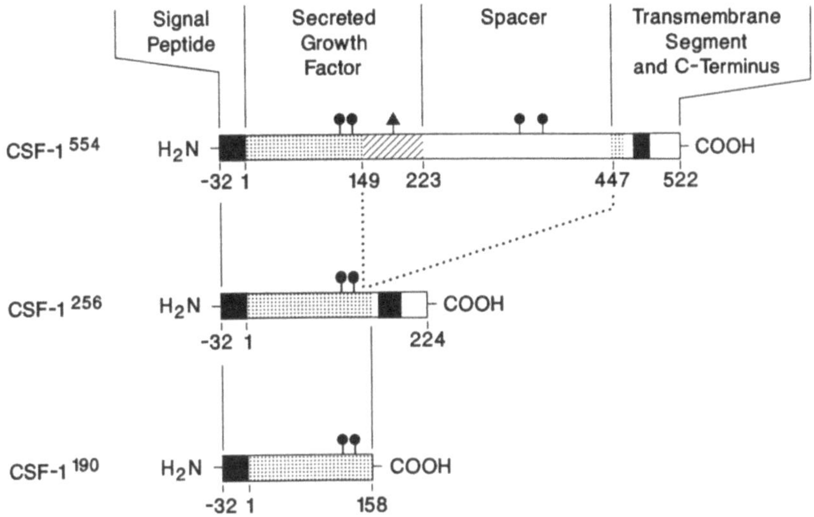

Fig. 1. Domain structure of CSF-1 precursors encoded by human cDNAs. The diagrams are derived from the amino acid sequences of CSF-1^{554} and CSF-1^{256} deduced from the nucleotide sequences of the 4 kb and the 1.6 kb clones, respectively. Amino acids are numbered beneath the corresponding line drawing such that the aminoterminus of the soluble growth factor (stippled) is indicated as position 1. The contiguous segment of 298 amino acids, present in CSF-1^{554} and absent in CSF-1^{256}, is delimited by dotted lines. Sequences from this unique coding region that are included at the C-terminus of the soluble growth factor processed from CSF-1^{554} are cross-hatched. Canonical sites for addition of N-linked oligosaccharides are indicated by closed circles. The secreted product derived from CSF-1^{554} also contains O-linked carbohydrate (closed triangle) for which the attachment site is currently not known. Shown at the bottom is a genetically engineered, carboxylterminal truncated form of CSF-1 which is 190 amino acids in length and lacks the membrane-spanning segment and C-terminal domain of CSF-1^{256}. CSF-1^{190} is the precursor to a biologically active, 158 amino acid growth factor generated after removal of the aminoterminal signal peptide.

aminoterminal signal peptide and the presumptive transmembrane domain. The soluble growth factor derived from the 256 amino acid precursor is a glycoprotein dimer of about 44 kilodaltons (kd), composed of 22 kd subunits that contain N-linked oligosaccharides (Csejtey and Boosman, 1986; Rettenmier et al., 1987). By contrast, the secreted product of the larger 554 amino acid precursor is about 86 kd and composed of 43 kd subunits. Part of the size difference between the two soluble forms of CSF-1 is due to the larger product having additional carboxylterminal amino acids derived from the unique coding sequence of the 4 kb cDNA (Wong et al., 1987). Moreover, the soluble 43 kd subunit encoded by the larger clones contains both N-linked and O-linked oligosaccharides, of which the latter are not present in the 22 kd N-glycosylated monomer derived from the 1.6 kb cDNA product (Rettenmier and Roussel, 1988; Manos, 1988). Removal of the carbohydrate yielded polypeptide chains of about 19 kd and 26 kd for the secreted forms of CSF-1 derived from the smaller and larger precursors, respectively (Rettenmier and Roussel, 1988). The latter result is in good agreement with the finding that the soluble growth factor derived by proteolysis of the 554 amino acid precursor is 223 amino acids in length (Clark and Kamen, 1987).

Also shown at the bottom of Fig. 1 is the structure of a truncated CSF-1 precursor which was generated by placement of a termination codon after amino acid 190 in the coding sequence of the 1.6 kb cDNA (Heard et al., 1987). Following cleavage of the 32 residues in the aminoterminal signal peptide, the biologically active product of the truncated clone is thus predicted to contain 158 amino acids (see below).

<u>Vector-mediated expression of human CSF-1 cDNAs</u>

Cloning of the human CSF-1 cDNAs into viral vectors has led to their expression in various cells and permitted the study of their encoded products by conventional biochemical techniques of radiolabeling and immune precipitation. Transfected murine NIH-3T3 fibroblasts expressing retroviral vectors containing either the 1.6 kb or the 4 kb clones produce biologically active human CSF-1 and are transformed by an autocrine mechanism when cotransfected with a human c-<u>fms</u> (CSF-1 receptor) cDNA (Roussel et al., 1987; Rettenmier and Roussel, 1988). Biochemical analyses of the products of both cDNAs revealed that the secreted growth factors were smaller than the corresponding cell-associated forms, suggesting that the soluble molecules were generated by proteolytic cleavage of glycosylated polypeptides. However, the two clones express different forms of soluble CSF-1 that are derived from their respective precursors by alternative processing mechanisms.

When murine cells expressing the human 1.6 kb or 4 kb CSF-1 cDNAs are metabolically labeled with [^{35}S]methionine in the presence of tunicamycin, an inhibitor of N-glycosylation, the cell-associated CSF-1 molecules are about 23 kd and 62 kd in size, respectively (Rettenmier et al., 1987; Rettenmier and Roussel, 1988; Manos, 1988). These molecular weights are in good agreement with those predicted from the cDNA coding sequences after removal of the aminoterminal signal peptide. In the absence of tunicamycin, the two cell-associated CSF-1 precursors undergo cotranslational addition of N-linked, high-mannose oligosaccharides to yield glycosylated forms of 32 kd and 70 kd, respectively. The 32 kd product of the 1.6 kb cDNA is converted to a 34 kd glycoprotein by processing of the N-linked carbohydrate to complex oligosaccharide chains (Rettenmier et al., 1987). However, only N-linked oligosaccharides of the immature high-mannose type are detected on the glycosylated 70 kd CSF-1 precursor encoded by the 4 kb clone (Rettenmier and Roussel, 1988; Manos, 1988). This probably reflects the more rapid rates of cleavage for the cell-associated 70 kd molecule and secretion of its soluble growth factor product (see below).

Early studies on the structure of CSF-1 demonstrated that disulfide reduction converted the soluble homodimeric growth factor to monomeric subunits and abolished its biological activity (Stanley and Heard, 1977; Das et al., 1981; Das and Stanley, 1982). Moreover, the CSF-1 precursors encoded by the human 1.6 kb and 4 kb cDNAs were assembled into disulfide-linked homodimers rapidly after synthesis in NIH-3T3 cells (Rettenmier et al., 1987; Rettenmier and Roussel, 1988). Thus, the molecular weights of the two cell-associated molecules under nonreducing conditions were 68 kd and 140 kd, respectively. Since corresponding unglycosylated homodimers of the two precursors were also generated in the presence of tunicamycin, the addition of N-linked carbohydrate was not required for dimeric assembly of these subunits.

The cell-associated CSF-1 precursors encoded by the two human cDNAs exhibited markedly different rates of turnover. Pulse-chase analyses by metabolic radiolabeling with [^{35}S]methionine demonstrated that the 68 kd homodimer encoded by the 1.6 kb clone had a half-life of about 4 to 6 hours and only low amounts of the soluble growth factor product were recovered from the culture medium (Rettenmier et al., 1987). By contrast, the larger CSF-1 precursor encoded by the 4 kb cDNA was rapidly turned over with quantitative recovery of the secreted growth factor within about 1 hour after synthesis (Rettenmier and Roussel, 1988; Manos, 1988). Thus, although both human CSF-1 precursors are cleaved to generate a soluble growth factor in this expression system, there appear to be differences in the mechanisms of processing that may have biological significance.

Cell surface expression of the human 1.6 kb CSF-1 cDNA product

The cell-associated 68 kd homodimer encoded by the smaller human cDNA is transported to the plasma membrane of transfected NIH-3T3 cells and subsequently undergoes proteolytic cleavage to release a soluble 44 kd CSF-1 dimer composed of 22 kd subunits (Rettenmier et al., 1987). CSF-1 epitopes were detected at the cell surface by flow cytometry with antibody to the secreted growth factor, and the 68 kd precursor was directly labeled on the plasma membrane of viable cells by lactoperoxidase-catalyzed radioiodination. Since surface epitopes of the 68 kd homodimer were shared by soluble CSF-1, the precursor is apparently oriented in the membrane with its N-terminal growth factor moiety exposed to the extracellular space and its short C-terminal domain in the cytoplasm. However, less than 10% of the membrane-bound CSF-1 molecules labeled at the cell surface were recovered as soluble growth factor in the culture medium, indicating that cleavage of the precursor and release of the product were not efficient in this system.

Similar results were achieved by introduction of the human 1.6 kb cDNA into other murine cell lines including C127 mammary carcinoma cells (Heard et al., 1987) and a growth factor-dependent macrophage cell line (Roussel et al., 1988). Thus, the smaller human cDNA directs the synthesis of a plasma membrane-bound 68 kd homodimeric CSF-1 precursor that is inefficiently processed to generate the soluble growth factor in several types of cultured murine cells.

When NIH-3T3 cells expressing the 1.6 kb human cDNA were incubated in the presence of trypsin, the 68 kd molecules on the cell surface were cleaved to 44 kd homodimers that comigrated in SDS-polyacrylamide gels with the soluble CSF-1 recovered in the absence of exogenously added protease (Rettenmier et al., 1987). The latter result suggests that the rate of release of soluble growth factor from the membrane-bound precursor might be regulated by trypsin-like proteases under physiological conditions, such as occur at sites of tissue injury.

<u>Role of the transmembrane sequence is demonstrated by a truncated CSF-1 precursor</u>

The segment of 23 hydrophobic amino acids near the C-terminus of the CSF-1 precursors was proposed to anchor these molecules in the membrane (Kawasaki et al., 1985). This model predicts that proteolytic cleavage must take place on the aminoterminal side of the transmembrane sequence to release the soluble growth factor. Site-directed mutagenesis was therefore used to place a TGA termination codon after amino acid residue 190 in the coding sequence of the 1.6 kb human cDNA (Heard et al., 1987). This mutant was predicted to encode a CSF-1 product of 158 amino acids after cleavage of the aminoterminal 32 residues of the signal peptide. The truncated molecule was biologically active for stimulating the growth of CSF-1 receptor-bearing cells and transformed NIH-3T3 cells when coexpressed with the human c-<u>fms</u> proto-oncogene product. Like the membrane-bound precursor encoded by the intact 1.6 kb cDNA, the prematurely terminated form underwent cotranslational addition of N-linked oligosaccharides and rapid assembly into disulfide-linked homodimers. However, the truncated molecule was not membrane-associated and was not detected at the cell surface. Rather, the product encoded by the mutant was directly and quantitatively secreted into the culture medium.

The polypeptide chain of the secreted molecule was the same size as its cell-associated form, suggesting that the truncated product did not undergo further proteolysis following removal of the aminoterminal signal peptide (Heard et al., 1987). Moreover, the glycosylated form of the truncated molecule was the same size as the soluble growth factor generated by proteolytic cleavage of the membrane-bound precursor encoded by the 1.6 kb cDNA, and removal of the N-linked carbohydrate confirmed that their polypeptide chains were very similar in length. These results indicated that the C-terminal hydrophobic segment of the full-length precursor functions as a transmembrane anchor sequence and cleavage of the plasma membrane-bound molecule takes place in the vicinity of amino acid 158.

<u>The product of the 4 kb CSF-1 cDNA is rapidly cleaved and efficiently secreted</u>

In contrast to the results with the product of the smaller cDNA, the cell-associated precursor encoded by the human 4 kb clone was efficiently cleaved to yield a rapidly secreted 86 kd glycosylated homodimer composed of 43 subunits (Rettenmier and Roussel, 1988; Manos, 1988). Although the 70 kd precursor was recovered as a membrane-bound glycoprotein with the expected orientation in the ER, neither the cell-associated precursor nor the soluble growth factor were detected on the plasma membrane (Rettenmier and Roussel, 1988). Whereas the smaller CSF-1 product encoded by the 1.6 kb clone contained only N-linked carbohydrate chains, digestions with glycosidic enzymes revealed that the soluble product of the 4 kb cDNA had both

Table 1. Properties of human CSF-1 cDNA products

Primary translation product	Size of the glycosylated cell-associated precursor [a]		Cell-associated form detected as a membrane-bound glycoprotein		Size of the soluble growth factor product (monomer subunit)		Glycosylation of the secreted growth factor molecule	
	Mol. wt.	Amino acids	Endoplasmic reticulum	Plasma membrane	Mol. wt.	Amino acids	N-linked[b]	O-linked[c]
$CSF\text{-}1^{554}$	70 kd	522	Yes	No	43 kd	(189)[d]	Yes	Yes
$CSF\text{-}1^{256}$	34 kd	224	Yes	Yes	22 kd	(158)[e]	Yes	No
$CSF\text{-}1^{190}$ [f]	21 kd [g]	158	No	No	22 kd [g]	158	Yes	No

a Following removal of the aminoterminal signal peptide of 32 amino acids.

b Oligosaccharides attached to asparagine residues at sites of canonical acceptor sequences (Asn-X-Ser/Thr).

c Carbohydrate chains attached to serine or threonine residues.

d Minimum estimate initially determined by amino acid sequence analysis of tryptic peptides (Wong et al., 1987). More recent studies indicate that the soluble growth factor has 223 amino acids (Clark and Kamen, 1987).

e Estimate based on the similarity in size to the soluble product derived from the truncated $CSF\text{-}1^{190}$.

f Biologically active molecule derived by placement of a termination codon after that for amino acid 190 in the sequence encoding $CSF\text{-}1^{256}$.

g The size difference between the cell-associated and secreted forms of the truncated product is due to processing of immature N-linked oligosaccharides of the high-mannose type to complex carbohydrate chains.

N-linked and O-linked oligosaccharide chains (Rettenmier and Roussel, 1988; Manos, 1988).

Removal of the carbohydrate from the secreted 43 kd CSF-1 subunits encoded by the 4 kb clone yielded a 26 kd polypeptide, as compared to an unglycosylated 19 kd monomer derived from the corresponding product of the 1.6 kb cDNA (Rettenmier and Roussel, 1988). The latter result is consistent with the observation that the carboxyl-terminus of the larger soluble product is derived from the unique coding sequence insert of the 4 kb clone (Wong et al., 1987), and recent findings have indicated that the secreted molecule derived from CSF-1^{554} is 223 amino acids in length (Clark and Kamen, 1987). Thus, the membrane-bound precursors specified by the two human cDNAs are differentially processed with respect to both the sites of proteolysis within the polypeptides and the subcellular locations where the cleavages occur. The properties of the various cell-associated and secreted forms of CSF-1 encoded by the full-length 1.6 kb and 4 kb cDNAs as well as the truncation mutant derived from the smaller clone are summarized in Table 1.

DISCUSSION

A physiological role for cell surface CSF-1?

The finding that the two human CSF-1 precursors undergo different post-translational processing events raises that possibility that they may serve alternative functions *in vivo*. Studies with the 190 amino acid product of a truncation mutant derived from the 1.6 kb cDNA demonstrated that the aminoterminal signal peptide and residues 1-158 of the soluble molecule are sufficient for biological activity. All of these forms of secreted CSF-1 stimulate the growth of receptor-bearing cells, and no differences in their physiological function have yet been documented. One hypothesis is that the efficiently secreted product derived from CSF-1^{554} is the major form of the growth factor released into the circulation, whereas the plasma membrane-bound precursor encoded by the 1.6 kb cDNA might be able to interact directly with receptor-bearing targets in circumstances involving cell-cell contact.

Surface expression of CSF-1 on cells producing this growth factor was first demonstrated by Cifone and Defendi (1974) who showed that trypsin treatment of mouse L cells released a biologically active macrophage growth factor identical to CSF-1 (Stanley et al., 1976). As described above, the product of the 1.6 kb human CSF-1 cDNA is expressed on the plasma membrane of murine cells where it is inefficiently cleaved to yield the soluble growth factor in several expression systems. The molecule is stably expressed at the cell surface in a form that binds a monoclonal antibody to CSF-1, suggesting that the growth factor domain of the membrane-bound precursor assumes a conformation similar to that of the secreted product. Indeed, preliminary studies indicate that the membrane-bound form of CSF-1 at the cell surface is biologically active (J. Stein and C.W. Rettenmier, unpublished observations). The mechanisms by which the soluble and membrane-associated forms of the growth factor might bind to and stimulate CSF-1 receptors are diagrammed in Fig. 2.

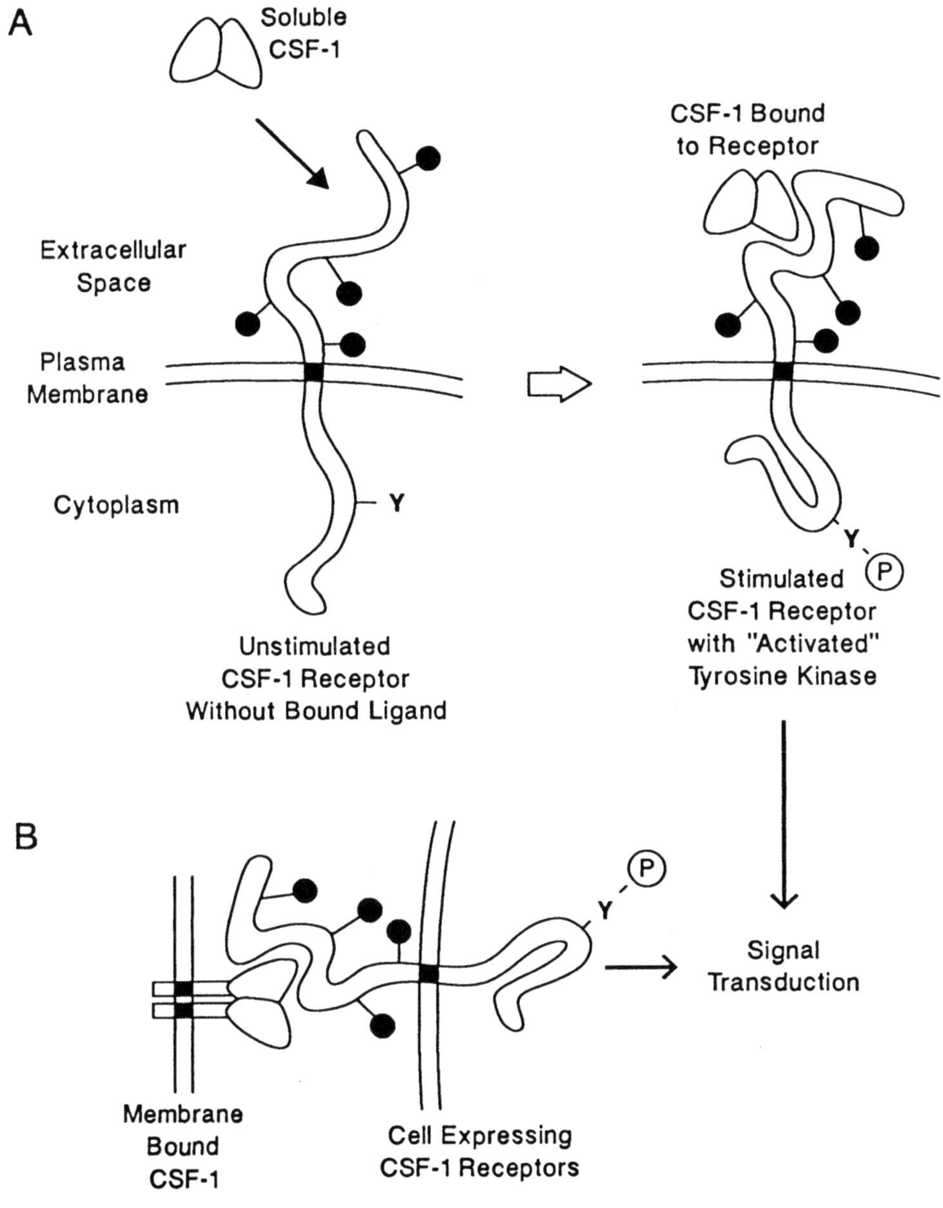

Fig. 2. Topology for binding of soluble (A) or membrane-bound (B) CSF-1 to its c-fms-encoded receptor. The interaction of the growth factor with the extracellular domain alters the conformation of the transmembrane receptor and activates its cytoplasmic protein-tyrosine kinase. This results in autophosphorylation of the CSF-1 receptor on tyrosine and phosphorylation of other cellular substrates, leading to transduction of the growth factor-initiated signal to the nucleus and thus altering patterns of gene transcription to effect the cellular response.

Further post-translational modifications and regulation of CSF-1 production

When culture medium from cells expressing the human 4 kb cDNA is incubated with antibody to CSF-1, the secreted growth factor is coprecipitated with material that migrates as a diffuse band of about 200 kd in SDS-polyacrylamide gels (Rettenmier and Roussel, 1988; Manos, 1988). This material has properties suggestive of a cellular proteoglycan that may bind the soluble 43 kd CSF-1 molecule in a manner analogous to that observed for heparin binding to fibroblast growth factors. The 200 kd material was not detected in association with the secreted 22 kd growth factor encoded by the full-length 1.6 kb clone or the soluble product of the truncation mutant. These results suggest that the secreted CSF-1 product of the 4 kb cDNA may be bound to the 200 kd molecule by some of its unique carboxylterminal amino acid sequences or its O-linked carbohydrate. Association of interleukin-3 or GM-CSF with heparan sulfate has been shown to be important for their ability to support the growth of bone marrow progenitors in a model of stromal cell-mediated hematopoiesis (Roberts et al., 1988). Similar interactions with components of the extracellular matrix may also play a role in the presentation of CSF-1 to receptor-bearing target cells.

Synthesis of CSF-1 mRNA is not always sufficient for the recovery of biologically active growth factor in experimental systems. For example, the 4 kb mRNA is the major CSF-1 transcript expressed under most conditions. However, in at least one inducible system, the production of biologically active growth factor is correlated with the appearance of smaller mRNAs (Ralph et al., 1986). Similarly, soluble CSF-1 was detected in the medium from human AML blasts expressing transcripts of its gene only when the cells were incubated in the presence of phorbol ester (Rambaldi et al., 1988). These results suggest that the production and release of CSF-1 might be further regulated by post-transcriptional or post-translational mechanisms in response to specific physiological inducers. A careful dissection of these events at the molecular level will be required to elucidate the controls for expression of this important biological response modifier.

ACKNOWLEDGEMENTS

The contributions of Drs. M.F. Roussel, J.M. Heard and C.J. Sherr to studies on the processing of human CSF-1 precursors are gratefully acknowledged. Work in the author's laboratory is currently supported by grant HL40603 from the National Institutes of Health and by the American Lebanese Syrian Associated Charities (ALSAC) of St. Jude Children's Research Hospital.

REFERENCES

Bartocci A, Pollard JW, Stanley ER (1986) Regulation of colony-stimulating factor 1 during pregnancy. J Exp Med 164:956-961

Cifone M, Defendi V (1974) Cyclic expression of a growth conditioning factor (MGF) on the cell surface. Nature (London) 252: 151-153

Clark SC, Kamen R (1987) The human hematopoietic colony-stimulating factors. Science 236:1229-1237

Csejtey J, Boosman A (1986) Purification of human macrophage colony stimulating factor (CSF-1) from medium conditioned by pancreatic carcinoma cells. Biochem Biophys Res Commun 138: 238-245
Das SK, Stanley ER (1982) Structure-function studies of a colony stimulating factor (CSF-1). J Biol Chem 257:13679-13684
Das SK, Stanley ER, Guilbert LJ, Forman LW (1981) Human colony-stimulating factor (CSF-1) radioimmunoassay: Resolution of three subclasses of human colony-stimulating factors. Blood 58:630-641
Downing JR, Rettenmier CW, Sherr CJ (1988) Ligand-induced tyrosine kinase activity of the colony stimulating factor 1 receptor in a murine macrophage cell line. Mol Cell Biol 8:1795-1799
Guilbert LJ, Stanley ER (1980) Specific interaction of murine colony-stimulating factor with mononuclear phagocytic cells. J Cell Biol 85:153-159
Guilbert LJ, Stanley ER (1986) The interaction of ^{125}I-colony-stimulating factor-1 with bone marrow-derived macrophages. J Biol Chem 261:4024-4032
Hamilton JA, Stanley ER, Burgess AW, Shadduck RK (1980) Stimulation of macrophage plasminogen activator activity by colony-stimulating factors. J Cell Physiol 103:435-445
Heard JM, Roussel MF, Rettenmier CW, Sherr CJ (1987) Synthesis, post-translational processing, and autocrine transforming activity of a carboxylterminal truncated form of colony stimulating factor-1. Oncogene Res 1:423-440
Horiguchi J, Warren MK, Kufe D (1987) Expression of the macrophage-specific colony-stimulating factor in human monocytes treated with granulocyte-macrophage colony-stimulating factor. Blood 69:1259-1261
Horiguchi J, Warren MK, Ralph P, Kufe D (1986) Expression of the macrophage specific colony-stimulating factor (CSF-1) during human monocytic differentiation. Biochem Biophys Res Commun 141:924-930
Karbassi A, Becker JM, Foster JS, Moore RN (1987) Enhanced killing of Candida albicans by murine macrophages treated with macrophage colony-stimulating factor: Evidence for augmented expression of mannose receptors. J Immunol 139:417-421
Kawasaki ES, Ladner MB, Wang AM, Van Arsdell J, Warren MK, Coyne MY, Schweickart VL, Lee MT, Wilson KJ, Boosman A, Stanley ER, Ralph P, Mark DF (1985) Molecular cloning of a complementary DNA encoding human macrophage-specific colony-stimulating factor (CSF-1). Science 230:291-296
Ladner MB, Martin GA, Noble JA, Nikoloff DM, Tal R, Kawasaki ES, White TJ (1987) Human CSF-1: Gene structure and alternative splicing of mRNA precursors. EMBO J 6:2693-2698
Lin H-S, Gordon S (1979) Secretion of plasminogen activator by bone marrow-derived mononuclear phagocytes and its enhancement by colony-stimulating factor. J Exp Med 150:231-245
Manos MM (1988) Expression and processing of a recombinant human macrophage colony-stimulating factor in mouse cells. Mol Cell Biol (in press)
Metcalf D, Nicola NA (1985) Synthesis by mouse peritoneal cells of G-CSF, the differentiation inducer for myeloid leukemia cells: Stimulation by endotoxin, M-CSF, and multi-CSF. Leuk Res 9:35-50
Moore RN, Oppenheim JJ, Farrar JJ, Carter CS Jr, Waheed A, Shadduck RK (1980) Production of lymphocyte-activating factor (interleukin 1) by macrophages activated with colony-stimulating factors. J Immunol 125:1302-1305
Oster W, Lindemann A, Horn S, Mertelsmann R, Herrmann F (1987) Tumor necrosis factor (TNF)-alpha but not TNF-beta induces secretion of colony stimulating factor for macrophages (CSF-1) by human monocytes. Blood 70:1700-1703

Pettenati MJ, Le Beau MM, Lemons RS, Shima EA, Kawasaki ES, Larson RA, Sherr CJ, Diaz MO, Rowley JD (1987) Assignment of CSF-1 to 5q33.1: Evidence for clustering of genes regulating hematopoiesis and for their involvement in the deletion of the long arm of chromosome 5 in myeloid disorders. Proc Natl Acad Sci USA 84: 2970-2974

Pollard JW, Bartocci A, Arceci R, Orlofsky A, Ladner MB, Stanley ER (1987) Apparent role of the macrophage growth factor, CSF-1, in placental development. Nature (London) 330:484-486

Ralph P, Nakoinz I (1987) Stimulation of macrophage tumoricidal activity by the growth and differentiation factor CSF-1. Cell Immunol 105:270-279

Ralph P, Warren MK, Lee MT, Csejtey J, Weaver JF, Broxmeyer HE, Williams DE, Stanley ER, Kawasaki ES (1986) Inducible production of human macrophage growth factor, CSF-1. Blood 68:633-639

Rambaldi A, Wakamiya N, Vellenga E, Horiguchi J, Warren MK, Kufe D, Griffin JD (1988) Expression of the macrophage colony-stimulating factor and c-fms genes in human acute myeloblastic leukemia cells. J Clin Invest 81:1030-1035

Rambaldi A, Young DC, Griffin JD (1987) Expression of the M-CSF (CSF-1) gene by human monocytes. Blood 69:1409-1413

Rettenmier CW, Chen JH, Roussel MF, Sherr CJ (1985) The product of the c-fms proto-oncogene: A glycoprotein with associated tyrosine kinase activity. Science 228:320-322

Rettenmier CW, Roussel MF (1988) Differential processing of colony-stimulating factor 1 precursors encoded by two human cDNAs. Mol Cell Biol (in press)

Rettenmier CW, Roussel MF, Ashmun RA, Ralph P, Price K, Sherr CJ (1987) Synthesis of membrane-bound colony-stimulating factor 1 (CSF-1) and downmodulation of CSF-1 receptors in NIH 3T3 cells transformed by cotransfection of the human CSF-1 and c-fms (CSF-1 receptor) genes. Mol Cell Biol 7:2378-2387

Rettenmier CW, Sacca R, Furman WL, Roussel MF, Holt JT, Nienhuis AW, Stanley ER, Sherr CJ (1986) Expression of the human c-fms proto-oncogene product (colony-stimulating factor-1 receptor) on peripheral blood mononuclear cells and choriocarcinoma cell lines. J Clin Invest 77:1740-1746

Roberts R, Gallagher J, Spooncer E, Allen TD, Bloomfield F, Dexter TM (1988) Heparan sulphate bound growth factors: A mechanism for stromal cell mediated haemopoiesis. Nature (London) 332:376-378

Roussel MF, Dull TJ, Rettenmier CW, Ralph P, Ullrich A, Sherr CJ (1987) Transforming potential of the c-fms proto-oncogene (CSF-1 receptor). Nature (London) 325:549-552

Roussel MF, Rettenmier CW, Sherr CJ (1988) Introduction of a human colony stimulating factor-1 gene into a mouse macrophage cell line induces CSF-1 independence but not tumorigenicity. Blood 71:1218-1225

Sherr CJ, Rettenmier CW, Sacca R, Roussel MF, Look AT, Stanley ER (1985) The c-fms proto-oncogene product is related to the receptor for the mononuclear phagocyte growth factor, CSF-1. Cell 41:665-676

Stanley ER, Cifone M, Heard PM, Defendi V (1976) Factors regulating macrophage production and growth: Identity of colony-stimulating factor and macrophage growth factor. J Exp Med 143: 631-647

Stanley ER, Guilbert LJ, Tushinski RJ, Bartelmez SH (1983) CSF-1 – A mononuclear phagocyte lineage-specific hemopoietic growth factor. J Cell Biochem 21:151-159

Stanley ER, Heard PM (1977) Factors regulating macrophage production and growth. Purification and some properties of the colony

stimulating factor from medium conditioned by mouse L cells. J Biol Chem 252:4305-4312
Tushinski RJ, Oliver IT, Guilbert LJ, Tynan PW, Warner JR, Stanley ER (1982) Survival of mononuclear phagocytes depends on a lineage-specific growth factor that the differentiated cells selectively destroy. Cell 28:71-81
Warren MK, Ralph P (1986) Macrophage growth factor CSF-1 stimulates human monocyte production of interferon, tumor necrosis factor, and colony stimulating activity. J Immunol 137:2281-2285
Wing EJ, Ampel NM, Waheed A, Shadduck RK (1985) Macrophage colony-stimulating factor (M-CSF) enhances the capacity of murine macrophages to secrete oxygen reduction products. J Immunol 135:2052-2056
Wing EJ, Waheed A, Shadduck RK, Nagle LS, Stephenson K (1982) Effect of colony stimulating factor on murine macrophages. Induction of antitumor activity. J Clin Invest 69:270-276
Wong GG, Temple PA, Leary AC, Witek-Giannotti JS, Yang Y-C, Ciarletta AB, Chung M, Murtha P, Kriz R, Kaufman RJ, Ferenz CR, Sibley BS, Turner KJ, Hewick RM, Clark SC, Yanai N, Yokota H, Yamada M, Saito M, Motoyoshi K, Takaku F (1987) Human CSF-1: Molecular cloning and expression of 4 kb cDNA encoding the human urinary protein. Science 235:1504-1508
Yeung YG, Jubinsky PT, Sengupta A, Yeung DCY, Stanley ER (1987) Purification of the colony-stimulating factor 1 receptor and demonstration of its tyrosine kinase activity. Proc Natl Acad Sci USA 84:1268-1271

The *ets* Family of Genes: Molecular Biology and Functional Implications

T.S. Papas, R.J. Fisher, N. Bhat, S. Fujiwara, D.K. Watson, J. Lautenberger, A. Seth, Z.Q. Chen, L., Burdett, L. Pribyl, C. W. Schweinfest, and R. Ascione.

Laboratory of Molecular Oncology, National Cancer Institute, Frederick, Maryland 21701-1013.

INTRODUCTION

To better understand the process of the cellular transformation and conversion of proto-oncogenes to the transforming retroviral oncogenes, our laboratory has pursued the study of the normal cellular genes comparing these to the homologous viral oncogenes. We have focused on the ets gene family which are related to sequences originally identified as a second cellular derived genes transduced by the avian leukemia virus, E26 (Watson et al. 1985). In mammals there are three ets genes located on two different chromosomes, termed ets-1, ets-2 and erg. The ETS-1 gene most related to the cellular ets captured by the virus (v-ets) is located on chromosome 11; the ETS-2 and ERG genes are located on chromosome 21. In higher mammals as well as humans these ets genes, are dispersed on separate chromosomes; but retain their homologous syntenic groups with respect to other genetic markers (Watson et. al. 1986). The ets genes are transcriptionally active, their gene products are homologous to one another and they are differentially regulated. Figure 1 presents a diagramatic comparison of the amino acid sequences of a wide variety of species ranging from Drosophila to humans. The predicted amino acid sequences from the nucleotide sequences illustrate that the homologous cellular-ets coding sequences have been conserved throughout metazoan evolution (Watson et. al. 1988 In Press).

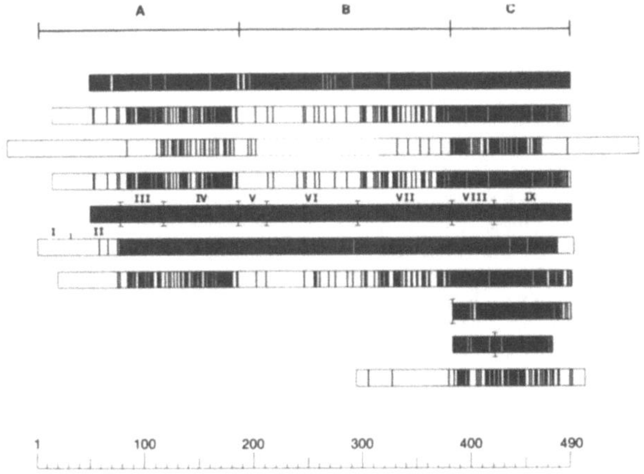

Figure 1. Comparison of ets-related Amino Acid Sequences.

Current Topics in Microbiology and Immunology, Vol. 149

The predicted ets proteins are compared to the chicken proto-ets-1 gene product since this gene is the one transduced by the E26 virus. The darkened areas represent regions of amino acid identity and the light areas are the regions of amino acid divergence. In the proto-oncogene we can identify three distinct domains. The carboxy terminal C domain is highly conserved in all the ets-genes we have characterized, with homologies >92% for the diverse animal species. The N-terminal 'A' domain is less homolgous showing only ~40% identity between Xenopus and human. The central region, domain 'B', shows the greatest divergence in mouse, human and Xenopus and is lacking in the ERG gene.

Expression of the ETS Genes

Having shown that specific regions of the ets-gene are highly conserved in insects, invertebrates and higher mammals, we have observed that ets-2 is expressed in a wide variety of proliferating cells, as well as in a model murine hepatic regenerating system (Bhat et. al. 1987) We observed that there is a transient accumulation of ets-2 messenger RNA during the early stages of liver regeneration. Also in the differentiating Drosophila and sea urchin developmental stages (Pribyl et. al. 1988, Chen et. al. 1988), the ets-2 expression reaches a maxima during early stages of embryo development. By contrast we have shown that the ets-1 gene was more highly expressed in the mouse thymus than in other tissue and the level did not change between 1 week and several months of age (Bhat et. al. 1987). To determine whether ets-1 and ets-2 gene expression could be detected in earlier stages of thymocyte development, we studied their expression in fetal, neonatal and young thymocytes (data not shown). The ets-1 expression coincides with the initial appearance of mature $CD4^+(CD8^-)$ thymocytes and is developmentally regulated. Thymocytes are a heterogeneous population of cells and therefore we decided to see if the ets gene expression corresponded to the appearance of specific subsets. We separated thymocytes into DN, $(CD4^-CD8^-)$, dLy-1,$(CD4^-CD8^-$low CD5), $CD4^+$ $(CD8^-)$, and $CD8^+$ $(CD4^-)$ subsets. The ets-1 mRNA level is about 10-fold higher in $CD4^+$ $(CD8^-)$ thymocytes than in the DN, dLy-1, or $CD8^+$ $(CD4^-)$ subsets (fig. 2).

Moreover, the level of ets-1 RNA found in unfractionated (UF) thymocytes could be almost entirely accounted for in the $CD4^+$ $(CD8^-)$subset. The ets-2 RNA was also found to be more highly expressed in the $CD4^+$ $(CD8^-)$subset (about 8-fold greater) than that found in the other three thymocyte subsets examined (Bhat et. al. 1988 In Press). Although both the ets-1 and ets-2 messengers were present in the $CD4^+$ $(CD8^-)$ subset, normalization of the mRNA amounts demonstrates that the ets-1 mRNA level is 10-fold higher than ets-2 in this subset. Thus, these results show that the elevated ets expression in $CD4^+$ thymocytes agrees well with our earlier results obtained from developing thymocytes (Bhat et. al. 1988 In Press). However, the expression of the ets-1 gene is much lower in peripheral $CD4^+$ $(CD8^-)$ T-cells as compared to $CD4^+$ $(CD8^-)$ thymocytes (data not shown).

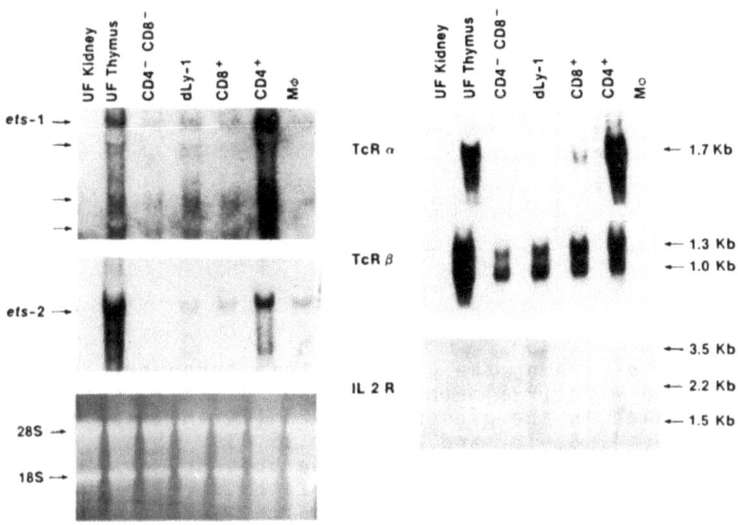

Figure 2. ets gene expression in thymocyte subsets: RNA blots (20 lg/lane) from UF kidney, UF thymus, macrophages (Mφ) and different thymocytes subsets were probed with specific probes. Transcripts detected by the probes are indicated on the left side. An ethidium bromide stained pattern of the RNA used to prepare blots is shown in the bottom left panel. Arrows below the ets-1 band indicates minor ets-1 mRNA species or ets-1 related mRNAs. Purity of thymic subsets as analyzed by flow cytometric analysis is as follows: $CD8^+$ cells: 99%, $CD4^+$ cells: 97.6%.

These findings implicates the ets genes involvement in thymocyte differentiation, or perhaps in the maturation of functional $CD4^+$ cells in order to provide helper/inducer functions. Because of the imporatant role that $CD4^+$ T cells have in the normal immune function, aberrations in the expression the ets genes may give rise to severe malfunctions in the immune system.

ets-2 is activated by protein kinase C

Using antisera raised against ets-specific peptides and proteins, we have shown that the human ets-2 gene product codes for a 56 KDa protein localized predominately in the nucleus and is phosphorylated (Fujiwara et. al. 1988 In Press). The protein is turned over very rapidly with a half-life of 20 minutes. The observed rapid turnover of the ETS-2 protein suggested that the expression of this protein is under precise cellular control. The modulation of its stability could quickly change the steady state level. We found that the elevated level of the ets-2 protein after stimulation of cells into tumor promoter 12-O-tetradecanoylphorbol-13-acetate (TPA) was due to decrease in the turnover rate of this protein (t1/2 2-3 hours) (fig.3).

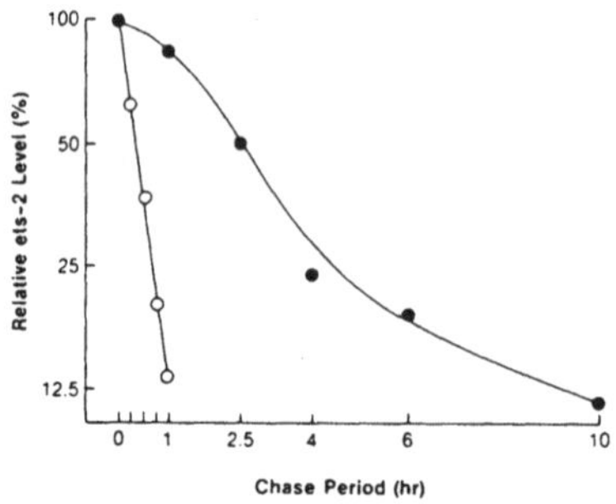

Figure 3. Effect of TPA on the ets-2 protein turnover. CEM cells were pulse-labeled with [^{35}S]methionine and chased in excess unlabeled methionine in the presence of TPA (10 nM). Cells were chased for 1, 2.5, 4, 6, 10, and 29 h, or 15, 30, 45 and 60 min. Decay kinetics of the ets-2 protein in the presence or absence of TPA. The X-ray film of the immunoprecipitates were analyzed by a densitometer and areas under peaks were calculated as measures of the amount of the labeled ets-2 protein. The labeled ets-2 protein levels at various chase periods were normalized to the 100% value obtained at zero time and plotted in semilogarithmic scale. The data was fit to a first order exponential decay curve with a correlation coefficient of 0.99. The open circles are control cells (t1/2=20 min) and the closed circles are the CEM cells chased in the presence of 10 nM TPA (t1/2= 160 min).

The stabilization of half-life by TPA is sufficient to account for most of the apparent increase (7-fold) seen in the ETS-2 protein (Fig.3). Collectively, the properties of the ETS-2 protein such as nuclear localization, phosphorylation, rapid turnover and response to Protein kinase C, indicated that this protein belongs to a group of oncogene proteins which are generally thought to have regulatory function in the nucleus (e.g., fos, myc, myb, and p53). It is known that Protein kinase C is involved in the transduction of signals mediated by a variety of hormones, neurotransmitters and growth factors (Fisher et. al. 1988 In Press). Physiologically, this enzyme is activated by diacylglycerol and Ca^{++}, both of which are generated by hydrolysis of inositol phospholipids triggered by receptor activation. Moreover, it has been shown that Protein kinase C is the receptor for the tumor-promoting phorbol ester, TPA, and its enzymatic activity is stimulated by the phorbol ester. Our results suggest further that Protein kinase C , either directly or indirectly, can regulate the level of the ets-2 protein by some specific post-translational mechanism. It can even be speculated that the stabilization of the ets-2 protein and the consequent transient elevation of its level, may be an intermediary step in the signalling process of the protein kinase C pathway, perhaps interconnecting this activation process with other proliferative gene(s) regulation. The deregulation or any subtle alteration of these controlling mechanisms may then, via the signal transduction pathway, cause a profound change in the intracellular physiology.

REFERENCES

Bhat NK, Fisher RJ, Fujiwara S, Ascione R, Papas TS (1987) Temporal and tissue-specific expression of mouse ets genes. Proc Natl Acad Sci USA 84:3161-3165.

Bhat NK, Komschlies KL, Fujiwara S, Fisher RJ, Mathieson BJ, Gregorio TA, Young HA, Kasik JW, Ozato K, Papas TS Expression of ets genes in mouse thymocyte subsets and T cells (submitted to J Immunol)

Chen Z-Q, Kan NC, Pribyl L, Lautenberger JA, Mourdrianakis E, Papas TS (1988) Molecular cloning of the ets proto-oncogene of the sea urchin and analysis of its developmental expression. Dev Biol 125:432-440.

Fisher RJ, Bader JP, Papas TS (1989) "In": Devita, Hellman, Rosenberg, eds. Oncogenes and the mitogenic signal pathway. Philadelphia. (In Press).

Fujiwara S, Fisher RJ, Bhat NK, Diaz de la Espina SM, Papas TS A short-lived nuclear phosphoprotein encoded by human ets-2 proto-oncogene is stabilized by protein kinase C activation. Mol Cell Biol (In Press).

Pribyl LJ, Watson DK, McWilliams MJ, Ascione R, Papas TS (1988) The Drosophila ets-2 gene: Molecular structure, chromosomal localization and developmental expression. Dev Biol 127:45-53.

Watson DK, McWilliams MJ, Lapis P, Lautenberger JA, Schweinfest CW, Papas TS Mammalian ets-1 and ets-2 genes encode highly conserved proteins. Proc Natl Acad Sci USA (In Press).

Watson DK, McWilliams-Smith MJ, Nunn MF, Duesberg PH, O'Brien SJ Papas TS (1985) The ets sequence from the transforming gene of avian erythroblastosis virus, E26, has unique domains on human chromosomes 11 and 21: Both loci are transcriptionally active. Proc Natl Acad Sci USA 82: 7294-7298.

Watson DK, Smith M, Kozak C, Reeves R, Gearhart J, Nunn M, Nash W, Fowle III JR, Duesberg P, Papas TS O'Brien SJ (1986) conserved chromsomal positions of dual domains of the ets proto-oncogene in cats, mice and man. Proc Natl Acad Sci USA. 82:1792-1796.

VI. Proposed Mechanisms in Myeloid Tumorigenesis

Adhesive Defects in Chronic Myeloid Leukemia

M.Y. Gordon, C.R. Dowding*, G.P. Riley, J.M. Goldman* and M.F. Greaves

Leukaemia Research Fund Centre, Institute of Cancer Research, Fulham Road, London SW3 6JB, United Kingdom
*MRC Leukaemia Unit, Royal Postgraduate Medical School, Hammersmith Hospital, Du Cane Road, London W12 0HS, United Kingdom

Normal human bone marrow contains a population of primitive haemopoietic progenitor cells that adhere to cultured bone marrow-derived stromal layers in vitro. These progenitor cells can be enumerated by a blast colony assay which is set up in several stages (Fig. 1; Gordon et al 1985a,b; 1987a).

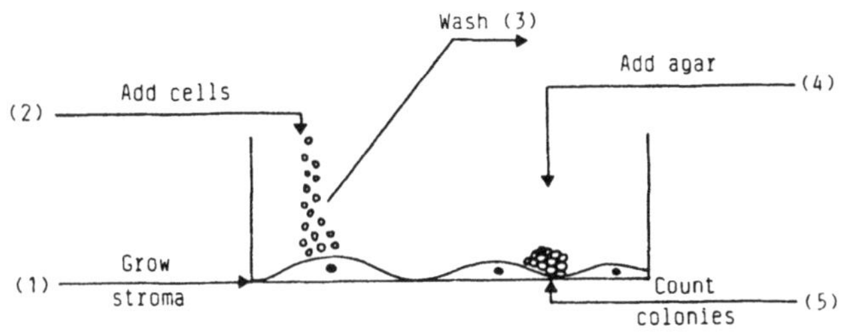

Fig. 1. Stages involved in the blast colony assay. Stages 1-5 are described in the text.

First (1), a stromal feeder layer is grown by plating $5x10^5$ normal human bone marrow mononuclear cells in 1ml of α-medium supplemented with 10% fetal calf serum, 10% horse serum and $2x10^{-6}$M methyl-prednisolone (MP) in 35mm petri dishes. The cultures are fed weekly by complete replacement of the medium, serum and MP until a confluent cell layer, consisting of fibroblastoid cells, fat cells and macrophages, covers the bases of the dishes and haemopoietic activity has disappeared. The non plastic-adherent fraction of $5x10^5$ fresh human marrow mononuclear cells in 1ml α-medium + 15% fetal calf serum is then added to the stromal layers (2) and they are incubated together for 2 hours. Any cells remaining in suspension are removed by vigorous washing (3) and cells that have adhered to the stromal layer are covered by 1ml of 0.3% agar in α-medium + 15% fetal calf serum (4). The cultures are then incubated for 5 days at 37°C in 5% CO_2 and colonies of 20 or more blast-like cells are counted under inverted phase contrast microscopy (5).

The introduction of a "panning" stage into the assay system meant that the efficiency of adhesion by different progenitor cells to a variety of surfaces could be measured (Gordon et al 1985b). In contrast to their efficient adhesion to stromal layers grown in the presence of

Current Topics in Microbiology and Immunology, Vol. 149

MP (MP^+), normal blast colony-forming cells do not adhere to MP^- (i.e. grown without MP) stromal layers (Gordon et al 1985b). Furthermore, committed progenitor cells (GM-CFC; BFU-E; Mk-CFC) do not adhere to MP^+ or MP^- stroma, suggesting that changes in adhesive properties are linked to haemopoietic cell maturation (Gordon et al 1985b).

There are no Bl-CFC in blood from normal individuals (Gordon et al 1985a) but numerous Bl-CFC circulate in patients with chronic phase chronic myeloid leukaemia (CML) (Dowding et al 1986). In these patients, the numbers of Bl-CFC in the bloodstream are linearly related to the elevation of the leukocyte count. The lack of Bl-CFC in normal blood indicates that an adhesive defect may be responsible for the exodus of Bl-CFC from the marrow in CML and may also lead to haemopoiesis in extramedullary sites. We have performed "panning" experiments with CML blood cells to test this hypothesis and found that CML Bl-CFC do not bind to stroma as efficiently as their counterparts in normal marrow (Gordon et al 1987b). Moreover, the CML Bl-CFC bind to MP^- stroma and form colonies whereas normal marrow Bl-CFC do not. Thus, it appears that CML Bl-CFC are less selective as well as less adherent than normal and these alterations could be associated with their capacities for extramedullary haemopoiesis and for circulation in the bloodstream.

Several explanations exist for the apparently reduced adherence to stroma by Bl-CFC in CML. First, the stroma may not provide sufficient binding sites for all of the Bl-CFC in CML blood. However, we have shown that a stromal layer can bind at least 2,000 normal Bl-CFC (Gordon et al 1987a) which is greater than the maximum (723/plate) measured in CML blood (Dowding et al 1986). Second, there may be two populations of Bl-CFC in CML (i.e. binders and non-binders) but we found that neither increasing the duration of coincubation of progenitors and stroma to 6 hours nor treating the cells with hydroxyurea to eliminate cycling cells altered the binding efficiency of Bl-CFC in CML (Gordon et al 1987b). Third, there may be a kinetic equilibrium between binding and detachment of Bl-CFC and stroma which is biased towards attachment by normal cell populations and which favours detachment in CML.

The latter possibility was suggested by preliminary results (Gordon et al 1987b) obtained when a third "panning" step was introduced into the experiment (Fig. 2).

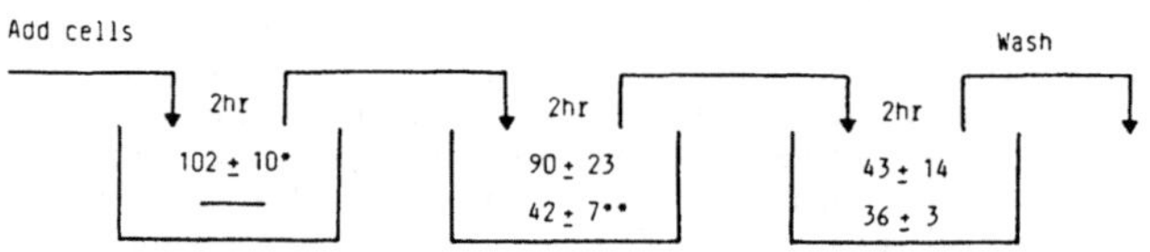

Fig. 2. Results of sequential "panning" of CML cells (from Gordon et al 1987b)
* Colonies per plate (mean ± SD of 3 experiments)
** Percentage transfer from one stage to the next

These results show that, whereas the numbers of colony-forming cells fell with sequential "panning", there was little difference in the proportion transferred from one stage to the next (cf. 42 ± 7 and 36 ± 3).

The experimental design shown in Fig. 3 was designed to test whether Bl-CFC in CML detach from stromal layers more readily than normal Bl-CFC. Plates in the different groups (A-D) are washed free of non-adherent cells 1-4 times at 2 hour intervals. Thus, any cells that detach during the two hours between one wash and the next will be progressively removed and unable to form colonies.

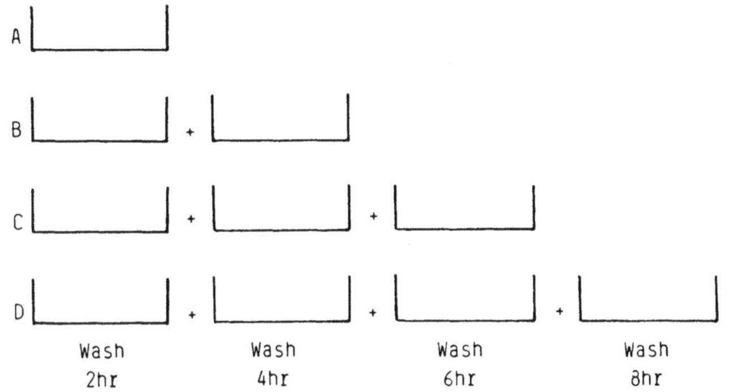

Fig. 3. Experimental design to measure rate of detachment of Bl-CFC from stromal layers.

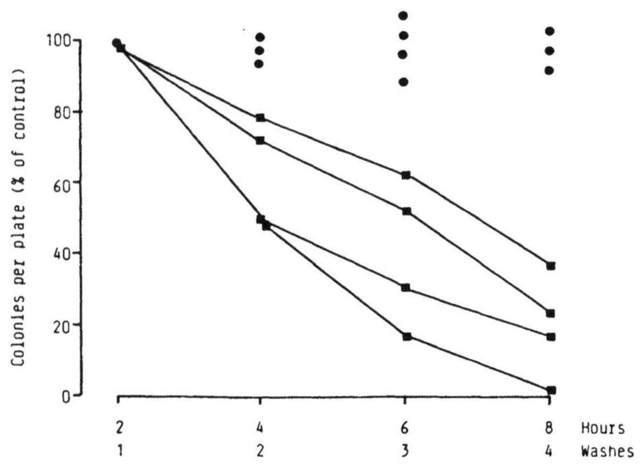

Fig. 4. The rate of detachment of CML Bl-CFC from stroma compared with the rate of detachment of normal Bl-CFC.
● Normal marrow Bl-CFC
■ CML Bl-CFC
Data points for individual CML patients are joined by solid lines.

Preliminary results (Fig. 4) have shown that CML Bl-CFC detach at a much faster rate than normal Bl-CFC. The numbers of colonies produced by normal cells in groups A-D (Fig. 3) are the same but the numbers of colonies produced by CML cells in group A are greater than in B>C>D.

The mechanism underlying the enhanced detachment from stroma by Bl-CFC in CML is unknown but possible explanations must consider a role for the increased c-abl kinase activity which is invariably associated with CML (Konopka et al 1985). Although the substrate for the kinase activity is unknown, it could be a cell surface or cytoskeletal protein involved in cell adhesion. We have tested the possibility that increased sialation of CML cells alters their adhesive properties (Baker et al 1985). However, prior treatment with neuraminidase did not significantly alter adhesion and colony formation by either CML Bl-CFC or normal Bl-CFC (Table 1).

Table 1. Effect of pretreatment with neuraminidase on adhesion by normal and CML Bl-CFC

	% recovery after "panning" on MP^+ stromal layers	
	No treatment	Treatment with neuraminidase
Normal Bl-CFC (n = 4)*	8 ± 2**	12 ± 3
CML-Bl-CFC (n = 4)	48 ± 5	32 ± 6

* n = number of experiments.
** Mean ± s.e.m.

Alternatively, since heparan sulphate is necessary for attachment by normal Bl-CFC (Gordon et al 1988), the production of a heparanase activity could account for increased detachment in CML. Enzymatic activities of this nature have been demonstrated in association with the metastatic behaviour of malignant cells and with the migration of normal cells (Matzner et al 1985; Bar-Ner et al 1985; Naparstek et al 1984). It is relevant also that phosphotyrosine-containing proteins may be concentrated in focal adhesion sites of normal cells (Maher et al 1985) and that the viral $pp60^{src}$ may be localised at sites of fibronectin degradation (Chen et al 1985).

REFERENCES

Baker MA, Taub RN, Whelton CH, Hindenburg A (1984) Aberrant sialation of granulocyte membranes in chronic myelogenous leukaemia. Blood 63:1194-1197

Bar-Ner M, Eldor A, Wasserman L, Matzner Y, Cohen IR, Fuks Z, Vlodavsky I (1987) Inhibition of heparanase-mediated degradation of extracellular matrix by non-anticoagulant heparin species. Blood 70:551-557

Chen W-T, Chen J-M, Parsons SJ, Parsons JT (1985) Local degradation of fibronectin at sites of expression of the transforming gene product $pp60^{src}$. Nature 316:156-158

Dowding CR, Gordon MY, Goldman JM (1986) Primitive progenitor cells in the blood of patients with chronic granulocytic leukaemia. Int J Cell Cloning 4:331-340

Gordon MY, Hibbin JA, Kearney LU, Gordon-Smith EC, Goldman JM (1985a) Colony formation by primitive haemopoietic progenitor cells in cocultures of bone marrow cells and stromal cells. Brit J Haemat 60:129-136
Gordon MY, Hibbin JA, Dowding C, Gordon-Smith EC, Goldman JM (1985b) Separation of human blast progenitors from granulocytic, erythroid, megakaryocytic and mixed colony-forming cells by "panning" on cultured marrow-derived stromal layers. Exp Hematol 13:937-940
Gordon MY, Dowding CR, Riley GP, Greaves MF (1987a) Characterisation of stroma-dependent blast colony-forming cells in human marrow. J Cell Physiol 130:150-156
Gordon MY, Dowding CR, Riley GP, Goldman JM, Greaves MF (1987b) Altered adhesive interactions with marrow stroma of haematopoietic progenitor cells in chronic myeloid leukaemia. Nature 328:342-344
Gordon MY, Riley GP, Clarke D (1988) Heparan sulphate is necessary for adhesive interactions between human early haemopoietic progenitor cells and the extracellular matrix of the marrow microenvironment. Submitted for publication
Konopka JB, Watanabe SM, Singer JW, Collins SJ, Witte ON (1985) Cell lines and clinical isolates derived from Phl-positive chronic myelogenous leukaemia patients express c-abl proteins with a common structural alteration. Proc Natl Acad Sci USA 82:1810-1814
Maher PA, Pasquale EB, Wong JYJ, Singer SJ (1985) Phosphotyrosine-containing proteins are concentrated in focal adhesions and intercellular junctions in normal cells. Proc Natl Acad Sci USA 82:6576-6580
Matzner Y, Bar-Ner M, Yahalom J, Ishai-Michaeli R, Fuks Z, Vlodavsky I (1985) Degradation of heparan sulphate in the subendothelial extracellular matrix by a readily released heparanase from human neutrophils. J Clin Invest 76:1306-1313
Naparstek Y, Cohen IR, Fuks Z, Vlodavsky I (1984) Activated T lymphocytes produce a matrix degrading heparan sulphate endoglycosidase. Nature 310:241-243

[illegible] of the marrow [illegible] [illegible]

[illegible] Suda T, [illegible] (198[illegible]) [illegible] [illegible] stromal [illegible] [illegible] [illegible]

[illegible] (198[illegible]) [illegible] [illegible] cells [illegible] [illegible]

Induction of Leukemia by Avian Myeloblastosis Virus: A Mechanistic Hypothesis

David Boettiger and Margaret Olsen

Department of Microbiology, University of Pennsylvania, Philadelphia PA 19104

INTRODUCTION

Avian myeloblastosis virus is the prototype virus for the myb oncogene. The virus was originally purified by Hall and colleagues between 1938 and 1941 by serial passage in chicken embryos (Hall et al.1941; Pollard and Hall 1942; Hall and Pollard 1943). In retrospect, it is clear that the original tumor tissue contained a mixture of viruses including Marek's Disease Virus, and avian leukosis virus. This contamination of virus stocks was a common problem in most of the early work due to the widespread distribution of these viruses in chicken flocks; so that even purified stocks became contaminated with other virus types when transferred to other laboratories (Johnson 1941). The strain A virus which Hall isolated induced a characteristic leukemia leading to death of the chicken in an average of 14 days post inoculation in about 80% of birds inoculated as embryos (Hall and Pollard 1943). The virus also caused similar disease in quail, turkey, pheasant, and duck (Pollard and Hall 1942; Hall and Pollard 1943), and appears to be identical to that induced by the current BAI Strain A propagated and studied for many years by Beard and colleagues (Beard 1963). The importance of this strain history is that there has been no change in the pathological phenotype generated by this strain, in spite of the some confusion with respect to the classification of the leukemic cell. The erythroblastosis associated with this strain (Johnson 1941; Beard 1963) was apparently due to a contaminant and was not observed by Beard or subsequent workers (Beard 1963).

PATHOGENESIS

In contrast to the majority of oncogene bearing retroviruses, the BAI strain A avian myeloblastosis virus (AMV) appears to transform only a very narrow range of cell types. Because of the confusion in analysis of the pathology of the disease in earlier work, we developed an in ovo model system in which 11 day SPAFAS chicken embryos were inoculated i.v. into a chorioallantoic membrane vein at an m.o.i. of >1 I.U./embryonic cell (.3mg of purified virus/embryo) (Olsen 1986; Olsen and Boettiger 1988b). The use of this high multiplicity for in vivo inoculation means that all susceptible cells become infected and transformed by the original inoculum and the progression of the disease does not rely on secondary spread. Hence the development of the pathology followed a protracted and highly reproducible time course. All inoculated embryos died prior to hatching (21 days) and exhibited a fulminant leukemia within 48 hr post inoculation. By 48 hrs. about 30% of the total blood cells in spleen, bone marrow, and liver were

Current Topics in Microbiology and Immunology, Vol. 149

leukemic cells. The progression of the disease is accompanied by anemia with the loss of red blood cells and by a stimulation of hematopoiesis which results in increased levels of immature cells of all hematopoietic lineages in the circulation (Olsen 1986; Olsen and Boettiger 1988a). It is likely that this increased hematopoiesis is secondary to the severe anemia. This could also explain some of the diagnostic confusion because of the presence of immature cells from unaffected lineages in the circulation. The blood picture in the embryo is similar to the disease in the adult (Durban 1980; Bonar et al.1959). The presence of large numbers of immature granulocytes led to the designation of the disease as a myeloblastic leukemia, since it was thought that the leukemic cells were the progenitors of these immature granulocytes (Beard 1963; Bonar et al.1959). However, this is not the case.

Examination of the developmental markers expressed by the leukemic cells (Durban and Boettiger 1981b; Ness et al.1987; Gazzolo et al. 1979) revealed the presence of macrophage markers rather than granulocyte markers. In the murine system activation of c-myb by retroviral insertion also gave tumor cells which a macrophage phenotype (Shen-Ong et al.1987). Induction of differentiation of the AMV leukemic cells with TPA resulted in a macrophage phenotype (Symonds et al.1984). And purified cultures of macrophages could serve as targets for transformation by AMV (Durban and Boettiger 1981a). However, we found that in vitro infection of cells derived from the yolk sac did not result in the infection of the granulocyte lineage cells (Olsen 1986; Olsen and Boettiger 1988b). They could, however, be infected using the in ovo model system described above. Following in ovo inoculation by AMV, yolk sac cells were removed and placed in vitro. By cell sorting and immunofluorescence >95% of the cells were infected and yet incubation in vitro led to the normal rate of granulocyte differentiation indicating that there is no effect of the virus on granulocyte differentiation and no evidence that infected granulocytes are able to transform despite the fact that they still divide 2-3 times in culture (Durban 1980; Olsen 1986). Hence the in vitro experiments were confirmed by the in ovo model system and demonstrated that the macrophage lineage is the only target for transformation by AMV in vivo as well as in vitro.

UNIQUE STATUS OF THE YOLK SAC MICROENVIRONMENT

The primary site of hematopoiesis in the 11 day chick embryo is the yolk sac. While quail-chick chimera transplants indicate that the majority of the hematopoietic stem cells at this stage are intraembryonic rather than in the yolk sac (Dieterlen-Lievre 1975), the yolk sac is the primary site for the expansion of hematopoietic progenitor cells and probably for the commitment to the specific hematopoietic lineages (Fig 1). The evidence for this comes from the analysis of the yolk sac cells for hematopoietic markers and morphology. Erythroid cells at all stages of differentiation may be identified; the remainding cells are of a blast cell type with no expression of markers characteristic of either the granulocyte or macrophage lineage (Durban 1980). When these cells are removed from the yolk sac and placed in culture, there is substantial differentiation into mature granulocytes reaching a peak at about 3 days and mature macrophages reaching a plateau level at about 5 days in culture (Durban 1980). The yolk sac cells are also susceptible to infection and transformation by AMV at the time of their removal from the embryo (Boettiger and Durban 1984). The susceptible population in the yolk sac can be purified from other cell populations using a Percoll density gradient. This population represents about 5% of the total yolk sac hematopoietic

Figure 1. Role of the Yolk Sac in Chicken Embryonic Hematopoiesis

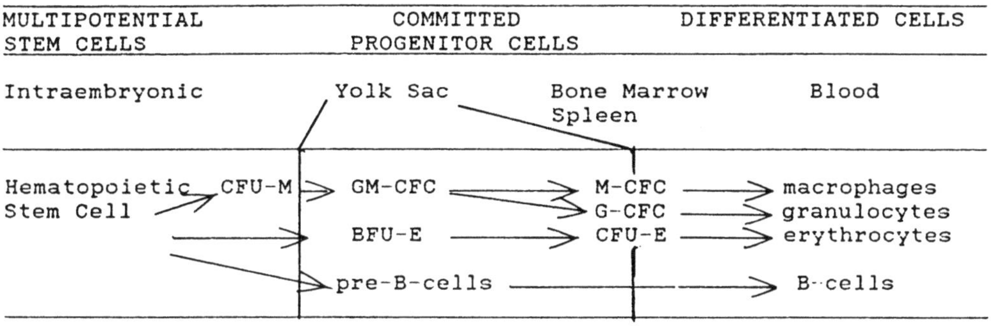

cells and contains all the macrophage colony forming units (Boettiger and Durban 1984).

Given this background of susceptibility of virtually all the yolk sac hematopoietic cells (except the red blood cells) to infection in the in ovo model, and the demonstration that infection of these cells in vitro led to rapid transformation of a specific sub-population, it was surprising to find a total absence of AMV leukemic cells in the yolk sac at all times examined following in ovo inoculation (TABLE 1). At this time all other hematopoietic tissues examined contained >30% leukemic cells. Is this absence of transformation explained by some property of the yolk sac microenvironment?

Table 1. AMV Leukemic Cells in Ovo

Gestation (days)	Organ	AMV Leukemic Cells Morphology	Colony Assay
13	Yolk sac	0%	0.07%
15	Yolk sac	0%	0.41%
13	Spleen	32%	0.94%
15	Spleen	45%	3.5 %
19	Spleen	69%	83.0 %
13	Bone marrow	37%	3.4 %
15	Bone marrow	51%	83.0 %

When these hematopoietic progenitor cells are removed from the yolk sac and placed in vitro, they undergo a single synchronous wave of differentiation and cells of the blast phenotype are no longer present after 48 hours. This suggests that the cells are competent to differentiate but that as long as they are retained in the yolk sac their maturation is blocked at a specific developmental stage. This fits with the absence of mature cells of the myeloid lineages in the yolk sac at any time in development from 9 to 17 days incubation (unpublished results). Focusing on the macrophage progenitors in the yolk sac, there are two properties which distinguish these cells from the progenitors found outside the yolk sac. 1) Separation of yolk sac cells on a Percoll gradient and probing for the expression of c-myb

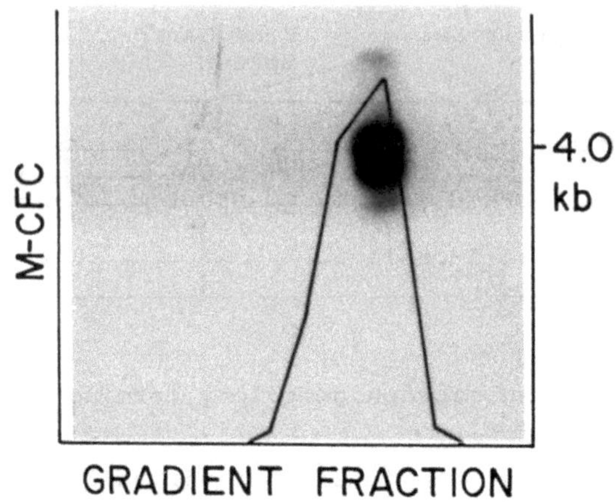

Figure 2 Northern analysis of Percoll gradient separated yolk sac cells probed for c-myb. Expression is in a single fraction corresponding to macrophage colony forming units.

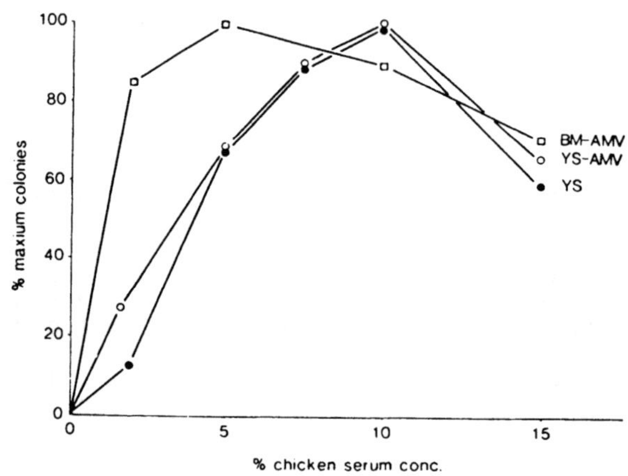

Figure 3. Dose-response curve for growth factor effects on colony formation of normal and AMV infected cells. Bone marrow □——□ ; Yolk sac (AMV infected) ○——○ ; Yolk sac ●——●

reveals a high level of expression which is restricted to this fraction. Figure 2 shows a northern analysis of this region of the gradient. The level of expression in this fraction is > 2 orders of magnitude above that expressed in the mature macrophage and 1 order above the levels reported in other situations or cell types with elevated c-myb expression (Klempnauer et al.1983). 2) Colony formation for either normal or AMV infected yolk sac cells requires higher levels of growth factor than in similar assays done on bone marrow derived cells suggesting that these cells represent an earlier compartment in the lineage than the progenitors present in the bone marrow (Fig. 3). The simplest interpretation of this data is that the yolk sac provides an environment for the proliferation of these hematopoietic progenitor cells but differentiation to a more mature stage requires release from the yolk sac microenvironment. If this is true, it implies that the yolk sac progenitors of the macrophage lineage are too immature to respond to the transforming action of v-myb, and express high levels of c-myb.

COUPLING OF DIFFERENTIATION AND TRANSFORMATION

When normal yolk sac cells are placed in culture and begin macrophage differentiation, there is a drop in the level of c-myb expression of about 2 orders of magnitude in the first 24 hours (Duprey and Boettiger 1985), which correlates with the decrease in the level of blast cells and an increase in a cell population which begins to express markers of the macrophage lineage. On the other hand, when yolk sac cells from in ovo inoculated embryos are placed in the same culture conditions there is very little macrophage differentiation, instead there is a rapid transformation. 21% of the cells in culture exhibit an AMV transformed phenotype with 24 hours and this raises to 42% by 48 hours. This includes the vast majority of the macrophage lineage cells from the original yolk sac population. A model for this differentiation process is shown in fig. 4.

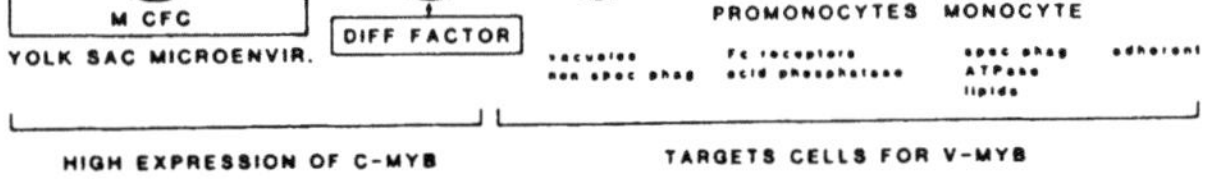

Figure 4. Model for the mechanism of myb function in differentiation and transformation.

The effect of the AMV infected yolk sac cells being released from the yolk sac microenvironment is that they are now free to differentiate but express high levels of myb. The effect of myb expression is to suppress the expression of most of the markers of macrophage differentiation (Durban and Boettiger 1981b). Hence these cells fail to mature and fail to reduce their division potential and rate. It is unlikely that myb expression actually increases the rate of cell proliferation since the cell doubling time measured both in vitro and in vivo (Durban and Boettiger 1981a; Beard, 1963) for the AMV transformed cells is about 3 days which is probably similar to or slower than that of normal cells with a similar level of phenotypic differentiation. This interpretation of the data suggests that the functions of c-myb and v-myb would be similar. The effect of the expression of either of these genes would be to suppress the expression of the differentiated cell phenotype and hence allow the cells to remain in a proliferative compartment. This is important for the expansion of the progenitor compartment prior to differentiation and restriction of proliferative potential, but it can lead to a leukemia when it occurs outside the normal constraints of the hematopoietic microenvironment.

PERSPECTIVE AND QUESTIONS

The model implies that c-myb would also be able to transform macrophage lineage cells. Data on this point is absent at present, however, correcting the single amino acid changes and deletion of the out-of-frame env sequences from AMV v-myb do not decrease its transforming potential (Stober-Grasser and Lipsick 1988). This still leaves the effects of both N and C-terminal truncation of the myb protein (Klempnauer and Bishop 1983) which need correction.

Elevated myb expression has now been observed in most hematopoietic cell types including T-cells (Sheiness and Gardinier 1984), B-cells (Bender and Kuehl 1986), and erythroid cells (Kirsch et al.1986). The promoter insertion activation of c-myb leading to B-cell tumors suggests that it may play a functional role in the B-cell, or at least in B cell neoplasia (Kanter et al.1988). The differentiation of erythroleukemia cells can be blocked by the introduction of a vector expressing c-myb (Clarke et al.1988), suggesting that c-myb could play a similar role in erythroid differentiation as postulated here for myeloid differentiation. In the other systems, it is not clear whether myb has a particular function or whether it's expression is neutral in the cell as it appears to be when v-myb is expressed in fibroblasts.

A number of laboratories have now reported the elevation of c-myb following mitogenic stimulation in both hematopoietic (Barka et al. 1986) and mesenchymal derived (Thompson et al.1986) cell types. The elevation of expression follows that of c-myc and appears to be transient. Hence it appears that the biology of myb will become considerably more complicated than suggested in the simple model based on the effects of v-myb and that it will be involved in processes in cell types outside the macrophage lineage. It is likely that these effects are usually obscured by the strong transforming effects of the AMV v-myb and the rapid death of the afflicted bird.

AKNOWLEDGEMENTS. This work was supported by grants from the National Cancer Institute.

REFERENCES

Barka T, Gubits RM, van der Noen HM (1986) Beta-adrenergic stimulation of c-fos gene expression in the mouse submandibular gland. Mol Cell Biol 6:2984-2989

Beard JW (1963) Avian virus growth and their etiologic agents. Adv Cancer Res 7:1-127

Bender TP, Kuehl WM (1986) Structure and function of c-myb proto-oncogene mRNA in murine B cells. Curr Top Microbiol Immunol 132:153-158

Boettiger D, Durban EM (1984) Target cell for avian myeloblastosis virus in embryonic yolk sac and the relationship of cell differentiation to cell transformation. J Virol 49:841-847

Bonar RA, Parsons DF, Beaudreau GS, Becker C, Beard JW (1959) Ultrastructure of avian myeloblasts in tissue culture. J Nat Cancer Inst 23:199-209

Clarke MF, Kukowska-Latallo JF, Westin E, Smith M, Prochownik EV (1988) Constitutive expression of a c-myb cDNA blocks friend murine erythroleukemia cell differentiation. Mol Cell Biol 8:884-892

Dieterlen-Lievre F (1975) On the origin of haemopoietic stem cells in the avian embryo: an experimental approach. J Embryol Exp Morphol 33:607

Duprey SP, Boettiger D (1985) Developmental regulation of c-myb in normal myeloid progenitorcells. Proc Natl Acad Sci USA 82:6937-6941

Durban EM (1980) Viral leukemogenesis: in vitro interactioned between avian myeloblastosis virus and differentiating hematopoietic cells. Ph D Thesis (Univ of Penn)

Durban EM, Boettiger D (1981a) Replicating differentiated macrophages can serve an target cells for transformation by avian myeloblastosis virus. J Virol 37:488-492

Durban EM, Boettiger D (1981b) Differential effects of transforming avian RNA tumor viruses on avian macrophages. Proc Natl Acad Sci U S 78:3600-3604

Gazzolo L, Moscovici C, Moscovici MG, Samarut J (1979) Response of hematopoietic cells to avian acute leukemia viruses: effects on the differentiation of the target cells. Cell 16:627-638

Hall WJ, Bean CW, Pollard M (1941) Transmission of fowl leucosis through chick embryos and young chicks. Am J Vet Res 2:272-279

Hall WJ, Pollard M (1943) Further studies on the propagation of fowl leucosis in chick embryos by intravenous inoculation. Am J Vet Res 4:287-293

Johnson EP (1941) Fowl leukosis - manisfestations, transmission, and etilogical relationship of various forms. Va Agr Exp Sta Tech Bul 76:2-21

Kanter MR, Smith RE, Hayward WS (1988) Rapid induction of B-cell lymphoma: insertional activation of c-myb by avian leukosis virus. J Virol 62:1423-1432

Kirsch IR, Bertness V, Silver J, Hollis GF (1986) Regulated expression of the c-myb and c-myc oncogenes during erythroid differentiation. J Cell Biochem 32:11-21

Klempnauer KH, Bishop JM (1983) Transduction of c-myb into avian myeloblastosis virus: locating points of recombination within the cellular gene. J Virol 48:565-572

Klempnauer KH, Ramsay G, Bishop JM, Moscovici MG, McGrath JP, Levinson AD (1983) The product of the retroviral transforming gene v-myb is a truncated version of the protein encoded by the cellular oncogene c-myb. Cell 33:345-355

Ness SA, Beug H, Graf T (1987) v-myb dominance over v-myc in doubly transformed chick myelomonocytic cells. Cell 51:41-50
Olsen, M. Differential effects of avian myeloblastosis virus infection on cells of the granulocyte and macrophsge lineages Ph.D. thesis, University of Pennsylvania, 1986.
Olsen M, Boettiger D (1988a) Pathogenesis of avian myeloblasatosis virus: an in ovo model. J Gen Virol (submitted)
Olsen M, Boettiger D (1988b) Infection of hematopoietic cells with AMV: A comparison of in vitro and in vivo targets. J Gen Virol (submitted)
Pollard M, Hall WJ (1942) Interspecies transmission of avian leukosis in embryos. Am J Vet Res 3:247-252
Sheiness D, Gardinier M (1984) Expression of a proto-oncogene (proto-myb) in hemopoietic tissues of mice. Mol Cell Biol 4:1206-1212
Shen-Ong GLC, Holmes KL, Morse III HC (1987) Phorbol ester-induced growth arrest of murine myelomonocytic leukemic cells with virus-disrupted myb locus is not accompanied by decreased myc and myb expression. Proc Natl Acad Sci USA 84:199-203
Stober-Grasser U, Lipsick JS (1988) Specific amino acid substitions are not required for transformation by v-myb of avian myeloblastosis virus. J Virol 62:1093-1096
Symonds G, Klempnauer KH, Evan GI, Bishop JM (1984) Induced differentiation of avian myeloblastos is virus transformed myeloblasts: phenotypic alteration without altered expression of the viral oncogene. Mol Cell Biol 4:2587-2593
Thompson CB, Challoner PB, Neiman PE, Groudine M (1986) Expression of the c-myb proto-oncogene during cellular poliferation. Nature 319:374-380

Role of Biologic Response Modifiers in the Growth and Differentiation of Myeloid Leukemic Cells

F. Ruscetti, G. Sing, P. Burke, F. Bettens, E. Schlick, S. Ruscetti and J. Keller

Laboratory of Molecular Immunoregulation, Biological Response Modifiers Program, NCI-Frederick Cancer Research Facility, Frederick, MD 217018*

INTRODUCTION

Human myeloid leukemic cells usually fail to grow or differentiate in vitro. The ability of cytokines to stimulate leukemic cell proliferation was first shown in well-differentiated T-cell leukemias using interleukin-2 (Poiesz et al., 1980). However, the role of hematopoietic growth factors in the initiation or progression of myeloid leukemic cells is not clear. A small fraction of almost all human myeloid leukemic cells show a proliferate response to one of these growth factors-IL-1, IL-3, CSF-1 GM-CSF or G-CSF (Griffin et al., 1986; Pebusque et al., 1988). These responding cells usually undergo terminal differentiation and cease cell proliferation. In rare cases, permanent cell lines which are usually factor independent can be established (Ferraro and Rovera, 1984). The question of why these hematopoietic growth factors can not control the growth and differentiation of leukemic cells remains unanswered. Making the assumption that the ability of these factors to transduce the correct biochemical signals was compromised in these cells, we asked whether differentiation signals that bypassed the cell membrane could stimulate terminal differentiation. In addition, since loss of responsiveness to growth inhibitors such as TGF-β has been proposed to contribute to neoplastic growth of various cell types, we examined the role of TGF-β in myeloid leukemic growth.

1,25 $(OH)_2$ D3 (1,25 Dihydroxycholecalciferol), a biologically active metabolite of vitamin D3, has been shown to be important for a functional immune system since deficiencies of vitamin D3 result in impaired immunity. These effects have been shown to be mediated by specific cytosol receptors for vitamin D3 were detected in lymphoid tissues. More recently, 1,25 $(OH)_2$ D3 was shown to influence hematopoietic cell growth and differentiation. It induces monocytoid differentiation of several human and mouse leukemic cell lines as well as normal human bone marrow cells (McCarthy et al., 1983). Besides, inducing differentiation, 1,25 $(OH)_2$ D3 also stimulates the functional capabilities of macrophages, including enhanced phagocytosis, antibody-dependent cellular cytotoxicity and transglutaminase activity. Also, phorbol-12 myristate-acetate (PMA) has similiar biological effects as 1,25 $(OH)_2$ D3 including induction of differentiation of the promyelocytic leukemia cell line (HL-60) along the monocytoid pathway and augmenting monocyte function. Retinoic acid, another biological with cytoplasmic receptors, has also been shown to stimulate differentiation of promyelocytic leukemic cells including HL-60 along the granulocyte rather than the monocyte pathway (Collins, 1987). The effectiveness of these molecules in stimulating variants of myeloid leukemic cell lines which can not differentiate in response to cell-surface acting factors was assessed.

* Department of Hematology, Johns Hopkins School of Medicine, Baltimore, MD (PB)
Laboratory of Genetics, National Cancer Institute, Bethesda, MD (SR)
Program Resources Inc, Frederick Cancer Research Facility, Frederick, MD (JK)

Current Topics in Microbiology and Immunology, Vol. 149

In addition to studying agents which limit leukemic cell proliferation through differentiation, there are strictly anti-proliferative molecules which may play a role in altering the development of leukemic hematopoiesis. The most interesting one is transforming growth factor β (TGF-β) which belongs to a family of proteins that regulate growth and differentiation of many cell types (Sporn et. al., 1986). TGF-β is a 25-Kd disulfide-linked homodimeric protein whose sequence is remarkedly conserved with only a single amino acid difference between mouse and man. Immunohistochemical studies using antibodies to the N-terminus of TGF-β1 showed that TGF-β1 is locally produced by cells in centers of active hematopoiesis (fetal liver and bone marrow). Platelets at 2 mg TGF-β/kg and bone at 0.2 mg TGF-β/kg are the two most abundant sources. These findings suggest that TGF-β is involved in regulating hematopoiesis. Results from our laboratory clearly demonstrate that TGF-β selectly inhibits the most immature (multipotent) hematopoietic progenitors but not the more mature (unipotent) progenitors are not affected (Keller et al., 1988; Sing et al., 1988). Hence, we examined the effect of TGF-β on leukemic cell growth.

METHODS

In general, two techniques are used to study the growth and differentiation of fresh hematopoietic cells and cell lines in vitro: (1) the measurement of cell number and type in suspension culture and (2) colony formation in semi-solid media by different cell types. Both assays depend on adding exogenous humoral factors for growth stimulation (Burgess and Metcalf, 1980). Factors used here include granulocyte-macrophage (GM-CSF), granulocyte (G-CSF) or macrophage (CSF-1) colony stimulating factors, which induce terminal maturation of the cell types for which they are named, and erythropoietin (Epo), which induces end-stage erythroid maturation. Also, interleukin-3 (IL-3), which induces multipotential bone marrow colony formation (CFU_{GEMM}) consisting of granulocytes, erythroid cells, monocytes and megakaryocytes, was used.

RESULTS

Effect of 1.25 $(OH)_2$ D3, PMA, and CSFs on Leukemic Myeloid Colony Formation

In order to be able to study the mechanisms by which these agents exert their differentiative effects, cell lines that could be differentiated by one or more of these agents were identified. WEHI-3B myelomonocytic leukemic cells were originally obtained from mineral-oil injected BALB/c mice. A differentiation positive (D^+) subline which terminally differentiates to granulocytes and/or macrophage in response to granulocyte colony-stimulating factor (G-CSF) (Burgess and Metcalf, 1980), whereas the differentiation (D-) subline has become hyperdiploid in karyotype, and can no longer differentiate in response to G-CSF (Ralph et al., 1976). Nicola et al., (1984) suggested that this occurred by alteration or loss of G-CSF receptors by D- cells. Thus, the ability of agents with cytosolic receptors to induce cell differentiation in WEHI-3B D^+ and D- lines was evaluated. Colony formation in the presence of purified CSFs of the three WEHI-3B variants, D^+,D- and D^+G, which preferently differentiates into granulocytes (Bettens et al., 1986), showed that in D^+ and D^+G cell cultures, G-CSF but not CSF-1 induces formation of differentiated colonies. This is accompanied by a reduction in number of colonies formed (Table 1). However, the D^- variant could not be induced to differentiate by any of the CSFs. The percentage of differentiated colonies composed of loosely dispersed cells which may or may not surround a central aggregate increased in response to CSFs in a dose dependent manner. In comparison to the effects of CSFs, stimulation of the same three cell lines with increasing concentrations of either PMA or 1,25 $(OH)_2$ D3 revealed different patterns of induction of differentiation. There is also a reduction in the total number of colonies formed. However, in response to PMA, dose-dependent formation of differentiated colonies was only detected for the D^+ subline whereas 1,25 $(OH)_2$ D3 induced dose-dependent formation of differentiated colonies in the D^+G and D^- lines. These data indicate that although the D^- line is unresponsive to normal hematopoietic differentiation factors, G-CSF or PMA, it still has the ability to terminally differentiate in response to agents that do not act via the plasma membrane such as 1,25 $(OH)_2$ D3 which has cytosolic/nuclear receptors. Vitamin D3 could act through different cellular pathways to induce differentiation or by bypassing only the first step of a common differentiation cascade used by agents with cell surface receptors. These results suggest that 1,25 $(OH)_2$ D3 may be useful in combination with hematopoietic growth factors (CSFs) as a therapeutic agent to induce leukemic cell differentiation in vivo.

Table 1. Differentiation of Wehi-3B Variants by Various Inducers

Cell Line	Differentiation Agent[a]	Total number of Colonies	% Differentiated Colonies[b]
WEHI D^+	-	147 ± 30	21 ± 6
	G-CSF	110 ± 19	95 ± 13
	CSF-1	114 ± 7	23 ± 4
	1,25 $(OH)_2$ D3	150 ± 29	27 ± 2
	PMA	73 ± 8	72 ± 2
WEHI D^-	-	145 ± 15	5 ± 3
	G-CSF	134 ± 12	10 ± 3
	CSF-1	138 ± 8	7 ± 2
	1,25 $(OH)_2$ D3	106 ± 38	73 ± 15
	PMA	116 ± 24	4 ± 2
WEHI D^+G	-	117 ± 37	7 ± 3
	G-CSF	83 ± 20	69 ± 4
	CSF-1	85 ± 18	16 ± 4
	1,25 $(OH)_2$ D3	80 ± 23	52 ± 10
	PMA	94 ± 16	17 ± 2

[a]The concentrations of the inducers were G, GM, M-CSF 1000 units, PMA 40 ug/ml and 1.25 $(OH)_2$ D3 1.6 ug/ml.

[b]Differentiated colonies consisted of loosely dispersed cells with or without a central aggregate. Results are expressed as mean ± SE of three experiments.

Effect of PMA and 1.25 $(OH)_2$ D3 on Myeloid Leukemic Cell Proliferation

As previously reported, terminal differential of myeloid leukemic cells is always accompanied by a loss in the ability to proliferate. The relationship betwween PMA or 1,25 $(OH)_2$ D3 induced differentiation and growth inhibition of the WEHI-3B lines was studied. For cell proliferation, ^{3}H-thymidine uptake was measured in liquid cultures. Stimulation of the three sublines with increasing doses of 1.25 $(OH)_2$ D3 inhibited growth as measured by thymidine incorporation. Concentrations of 0.4 ng/ml resulted in reductions of 75% and 50% reduction in ^{3}H-Tdr uptake in D^+G and D^- cultures respectively. Whereas the same concentration of 1,25 $(OH)_2$ D3 induced only a 5% inhibition of ^{3}H-Tdr uptake in D^+ cell cultures. On the other hand, PMA reduced ^{3}H-thymidine uptake by D^+ cells only. In addition, these results emphasize the ability of cells, which fail to respond to other signals, to be sensitive to 1,25 $(OH)_2$ D3 treatment with doses as low as 0.1 to 0.8 ng/ml. As a result of the inhibition of cell growth data, daily determination of cell numbers in samples from suspension cultures were performed. In 1.25 $(OH)_2$ D3 stimulated cultures, cell counts (expressed as a percent of counts determined in parallel untreated cultures) were reduced. Highest reductions were seen in D^+ and D^+G cell cultures. Cell numbers progressively decreased with incubation time, suggesting that 1.25 $(OH)_2$ D3 induced growth inhibition was not an acute effect on cell division but due to progressively reduced cell proliferation. PMA, which only affected cell multiplication of the D^+ subline, induced reduced cell counts in this cell line to about the same extent as 1,25 $(OH)_2$ D3 in the D^- cell line (15-20%) compared untreated cultures after 2-4 days of incubation). Thus, PMA effects cell growth over a shorter time period as compared to 1.25 $(OH)_2$ D3. For both agents used at concentrations not effecting cell viability, the maximum reduction in cell proliferation was seen after 120 hours. Longer periods of incubation did not increase the effects suggesting that in both cases some cells could escape the induced growth inhibition.

Granulocyte and Macrophage Differentiation of WEHI-3B Sublines.

To further show that growth inhibition was directly correlated with phenotypic differentiation of the cells, samples of cell cultures treated with differentiation agents, were removed to prepare cytospin smears which were then stained with Wright-Giemsa or used for AS-D chloroacetate esterase, α-naphtyl-acetate esterase and myeloperoxidase determination. As seen Table 2, increasing numbers of polymorphonuclear cells were detected in D^- and D^+G cell cultures treated with 1.25 $(OH)_2$ D3 reaching peaks values of 50-70% granulocytes. Whereas cells of the monocyte-macrophage lineage were identified in D^+ cell cultures stimulated with PMA. The observed morphological changes were supported by the histochemical staining of cells after treatment with various agents. Both chloroacetate esterase and myeloperoxidase, two stains specific for the granulocytic lineage are markedly increased in the D^- and D^+G after treatment with 1,25 $(OH)_2$ D3. To a lesser extent, some α-naphtylacetate esterase positivity which is a monocyte/macrophage specific marker was also seen in the 1,25 $(OH)_2$ D3 treated cells while the PMA stimulated D cultures were only positive for non-specific esterase. Thus, 1,25 $(OH)_2$ D3 was able to induce differentiation of myeloid leukemia cells unresponsive to G-CSF or PMA and, in contrast to PMA which stimulates responsive myeloid leukemic cells to undergo only monocytoid differentiation, 1,25 $(OH)_2$ D3 can induce granulocyte as well as monocyte differentiation in responsive cell lines.

Table 2. Differentiation of Wehi-3B Variants in Suspension Cultures

Cell Line	Differentiation Agent[a]	Myeloblast Promyelocyte Myelocyte[b]	Metamyelocyte Polymorphs	Promonocytes Monocytes
WEHI D^+	-	82%	18%	0%
	G-CSF	14	18	64
	PMA	31	0	62
	1.25 $(OH)_2$ D3	72	34	4
WEHI D^-	-	79	21	0
	G-CSF	73	4	23
	PMA	77	23	0
	1.25 $(OH)_2$ D3	45	50	5
WEHI D^+G	-	76	22	2
	G-CSF	25	56	17
	PMA	68	25	7
	1.25 $(OH)_2$ D3	28	72	0

[a] The concentrations of the inducers were PES 1:16 serum dilution, PMA 40 ug/ml and 1,25 $(OH)_2$ D3 1.6 ug/ml.

[b] Results are expressed as percent positive cells counted out of 1000 cells stained with Wright-Giemsa after 4 days of incubation with indicated agents or medium alone.

Effect of TGF-β on the Growth of Murine Leukemic Cell Lines

Since differentiation agents also cause a profound depression of cell growth, studies were undertaken to determine the effects of anti-proliferative agents on leukemic cell growth. TGF-β1 is a potent inhibitor of IL-3 induced murine bone marrow proliferation and colony formation but, surprisingly, has little or no effect on the growth and differentiation induced by GM-CSF, G-CSF or CSF-1. TGF-β1 also inhibits early erythroid differentiation stimulated by Epo in the GEMM assay while Epo-induced terminal erythroid differentiation is unaffected. Also, IL-3 but not GM-CSF induced granulocyte-macrophage colonies were inhibited. However, small clusters (5-20 cells) of terminally differentiated pure myeloid colonies were consistently seen in cultures containing IL-3 and TGF-β1. These results suggest that TGF-β1 selectively inhibits early murine hematopoietic progenitor growth and differentiation but not more mature progenitors (Keller et al., 1988).

Since these data suggest that TGF-β has a role in regulating hematopoietic cell progenitor populations, a variety of IL-3 dependent progenitor cell lines which represent leukemic myeloid cells blocked at various stages of differentiation based on phenotype, function, and morphology were tested for their sensitivity to TGF-β. In all cases tested, TGF-β1 inhibits the growth of IL-3 induced cell lines such as FDC-P1 and DA-1 (Table 3). The effective dose that resulted in 50% of maximal inhibition (ED-50) was simliar for all cell lines. This inhibitory effect was consistently observed among other IL-3 dependent cell lines regardless of their derivation. In addition to responding to IL-3, one cell line, NSF-60, proliferates in response to GM-CSF, CSF-1, G-CSF, IL-4, and IL-6. Growth factor-induced proliferation of NFS-60 is also inhibited by TGF-β1 in a dose-dependent manner with ED-50's of 6-10 pM. Since normal marrow cell growth and differentiation stimulated by GM-CSF and G-CSF were not inhibited by TGF-β, these results with NSF-60 suggest that the state of differentiation of a cell and not the growth factor responsiveness determines whether TGF-β will have an inhibitory effect. This is further supported by results obtained using factor independent cell lines. If these cell lines are made factor independent by transfecting oncogenes such as v-abl, v-src or v-fms into the cells, the cells remain as sensitive to growth inhibition by TGF-β as the factor dependent parent. In contrast, factor-independent leukemic cells of macrophage (P388D1, J774A.1), erythroid (TP-3, DS-19) or mast cell (P-185) derivation were not responsive to TGF-β (Table 3).

Table 3. Effect of TGF-β on Proliferation of Myeloid Leukemic Cell Lines

Cells	Stimulator(s)	TGF-β1 Inhibition [ED-50 (pM)]	Maximal Inhibition (%)
FDC-P1	IL-3, GM-CSF	8-24	80-90
B6 Sut A	IL-3	15-20	60-80
DA-1	IL-3	10-20	70-80
32D cl 23	IL-3	8-16	70-80
NFS-60	IL-3, GM-CSF, IL-4 G-CSF, CSF-1	10-60	60-70
NFS-vAbl	none	10-50	70-80
WEHI-3B	none	10-20	70-80
P388D1	none	0	0
J774A.1	none	0	0
TP-3	none	0	0
DS-19	none	0	0
P-185	none	0	0
Bone marrow	IL-3	10-20	40-60
Bone Marrow	GM-CSF, G-CSF	none	none

Effect of TGF-β on Fresh and Cultured Human Leukemic Cells

In order to test the effects of TGF-β on the proliferation of human leukemic cells, peripheral blood cells from 5 patients with untreated CML and 5 patients with untreated AML were cultured with 10 ng/ml of purified GM-CSF or G-CSF in the presence or absence of varying concentrations of TGF-β. As shown in Table 4, GM-CSF induced proliferation of leukemic cells could be inhibited by TGF-β in a dose-dependent manner with maximmal inhibition of 40-45% for CML and 60-70% for AML observed at 5 ng/ml of TGF-β. The responding cells were leukemic cells and not normal peripheral blood cells (PBL) since normal PBL do not respond to GM-CSF very well and more than 90% of the proliferating CML cells possessed the Philadelphia chromosome as determined by karyotypic analysis. Also, in contrast to normal bone marrow cells, the proliferation of CML and AML cells in response to G-CSF was also inhibited by TGF-β in a dose dependent manner (Table 4). However, in all cases studied, there was a certain amount of both autonomous and growth factor induced cell proliferation which was insensitive to inhibitory effects of TGF-β, suggesting that some fraction of the cells had escaped the regulation by TGF-β. To determine whether escape from negative regulation routinely occurred and whether TGF-β showed selectivity with regard to lineage specificity, human leukemic cell lines from the monocytic, myeloid and erythroid series were tested. All three erythroid cell lines (OC-1, K562 and HEL) showed little or no inhibition by TGF-β (Table 4). In contrast, the monocytic cell lines (U937 and THP-1) were both strongly inhibited by TGF-β. In addition, TGFβ strongly inhibited the growth of KG-1, a myeloblastic cell line while the more differentiated promyelocytic cell line was uneffected supporting the concept that sensitivity to inhibition by TGF-β is dependent on the differentiated state of the cell.

Table 4. Effect of TGF-β on Proliferation of Human Myeloid Leukemic Cells

Cells	Stimulator(s)	TGF-β1 Inhibition [ED-50 (pM)]	Maximal Inhibition (%)
CML	GM-CSF	5-15	40-50
CML	G-CSF	5-15	30-40
AML	GM-CSF	5-20	60-70
AML	G-CSF	5-20	40-60
U937	none	16-24	60-70
THP-1	none	16-24	45-60
KG-1	none	12-16	70-80
HL-60	none	0	0
OC-1	none	0	0
K-562	none	0	0
HEL	none	24	10-20
Bone marrow	GM-CSF	5-20	40-60
Bone Marrow	G-CSF	none	none

REFERENCES

Bettens, F., Schlick, E., Farrar, W., Ruscetti, F. (1986) 1,25 dihydroxycholecalciferol-induced differentiation of myelomonocytic leukemic cells unresponsive to colony-stimulating factors and phorbol esters. J. Cell. Physiol. 129:295-302.
Burgess AW, Metcalf D (1980). The nature and action of granulocyte-macrophage colony stimulating factors. Blood 56:947.
Collins, S. (1987) The HL-60 promyelocytic leukemia cell line: proliferation, differentiation and cellular oncogene expression. Blood 70:1233-1241.
Ferrero, D., Rovera, G. (1984) Human leukemic cell lines. Clin. Hematol. 13: 1461-1484.
Griffin, J., Younf, D., Hermann, F., Wiper, D., Wagner, K., Sabbath, K. (1986) Effect of recombinant GM-CSF on proliferation of clonogenic cells in acute myelogenous leukemia. Blood 67:1448-1455.
Keller JR, Mantel C, Sing G, Ellingsworth LE, Ruscetti SK, Ruscetti FW (1988) Transforming growth factor β1 selectively regulates early murine hematopoietic progenitors and inhibits the growth of IL-3 dependent myeloid leukemia cell lines. J. Exp. Med. 168:737-750, 1988.
McCarthy, D., San Miguel, J., Freake, H., Green, P., Zola, H., Catovsky, D., Goldman, J. (1983) 1,25 Dihydroxyvitamin D3 inhibits proliferation of human promyelocytic leukaemia (HL-60) cells and induces monocytic-macrophage differentiation in HL-60 and normal human bone marrow cells. Leukemia Res., 7:51-55.
Nicola, N. A., and D. Metcalf (1984) Binding of the differentiation-inducer, granulocyte-colony stimulating factor to responsive but not unresponsive leukemic cell lines. Proc. Natl. Acad. Sci. U.S.A., 81: 3765-3769.
Pebusque, M., Lopez, M., Torres, H., Carotti, A., Guibert, L., Mannoni, P (1988) Growth response of human myeloid leukemic cells to colony stimulating factors Exp. Hematol. 16:360-366.
Poiesz, B., Ruscetti, F., Mier, J., Woods, A., Gallo, R. (1980) T-cell lines established from human T-cell lymphocytic neoplasia by direct response to T-cell growth factor. Proc. Natl. Acad. Sci. USA 77:6815-6819.
Ralph, P., Moore, M. A. S. and Nilsson, K (1976) Lysozyme synthesis by established human and murine histiocytic lymphoma cell lines. J. Exp. Med., 143: 1528-1533.
Sing G, Keller JR, Ellingworth LE, Ruscetti FW (1988) Transforming Growth Factor β selectively inhibits normal and leukemic human bone marrow growth in vitro. Blood 72:1504-1509, 1988
Sporn MB, Roberts AB, Lalage MW, Assoian MA, (1986) Transforming growth factor-β: Biological function and chemical structure. Science 233:532.

MIX
Papier aus verantwortungsvollen Quellen
Paper from responsible sources
FSC® C105338

If you have any concerns about our products,
you can contact us on
ProductSafety@springernature.com

In case Publisher is established outside the EU,
the EU authorized representative is:
Springer Nature Customer Service Center GmbH
Europaplatz 3, 69115 Heidelberg, Germany

Printed by Libri Plureos GmbH
in Hamburg, Germany